Fighting Fatigue in
Multiple Sclerosis

FIGHTING FATIGUE IN MULTIPLE SCLEROSIS

PRACTICAL WAYS TO CREATE NEW HABITS AND INCREASE YOUR ENERGY

NANCY LOWENSTEIN, OTR

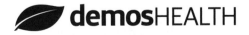

demosHEALTH

NEW YORK

Visit our web site at www.demosmedpub.com

Library of Congress Cataloging-in-Publication Data

Lowenstein, Nancy A., 1953-
    Fighting fatigue in multiple sclerosis : practical ways to create new habits and increase your energy / Nancy Lowenstein.
        p. cm.
    Includes index.
    ISBN-13: 978-1-932603-75-0 (pbk. : alk. paper)
    ISBN-10: 1-932603-75-1 (pbk. : alk. paper)
        1. Multiple sclerosis—Popular works.   2. Multiple sclerosis—Exercise therapy t—Popular works.   3. Fatigue—Popular works. I. Title.
    RC377.L69   2009
    616.8'34—dc22

                                                    2008046920

Special discounts on bulk quantities of Demos Medical Publishing books are available to corporations, professional associations, pharmaceutical companies, health care organizations, and other qualifying groups. For details, please contact:

Special Sales Department
Demos Medical Publishing
386 Park Avenue South, Suite 301
New York, NY 10016
Phone: 800–532–8663 or 212–683–0072
Fax: 212–683–0118
E-mail: orderdept@demosmedpub.com

Printed in Canada

09 10 11 12   5 4 3 2 1

CONTENTS

FOREWORD

Fatigue is a major problem in multiple sclerosis, affecting as many as 90% of individuals with the disease. It is most commonly defined as a sense of exhaustion and is often solely attributed to just mood or impaired physical functioning. Yet, fatigue is a symptom in its own right. Pharmacologic management is usually quite incomplete in solving the problem and non-pharmacologic interventions are critically important. When fatigue is not addressed it can lead to tremendous frustration and adversely affects quality of life for the person with multiple sclerosis, the family and health care provider.

In this wonderfully practical and highly individualized approach to fatigue, a very important management strategy is laid out in a detailed manner. Such an approach is critical for a symptom which causes such diverse problems. The specific recommended guidelines can lead to a dramatic improvement but will require individuals to be highly motivated and conscientious. Fortunately, the vast majority of individuals with multiple sclerosis have just this type of motivation and wish to improve their lives and reach their maximum potential. As outlined in this book, the key is to control the disease rather that be controlled by it. Fatigue can be effectively treated and this guide can provide the way. The step by step approach addresses fatigue head on and provides the necessary tools to overcome this pervasive symptom.

Lauren B. Krupp, MD

Professor of Neurology and Psychology at the State University of New York at Stony Brook and Medical Center, co-director of the adult MS Center at Stony Brook, and author of Fatigue in Multiple Sclerosis: A Guide to Diagnosis and Management

PREFACE

This book came about due to my 10 years working at the Mount Auburn Hospital Comprehensive Multiple Sclerosis Care Center where I have taught energy conservation techniques to people living with multiple sclerosis. I have done many presentations and workshops for the New England Chapter of the National Multiple Sclerosis Society on fatigue management. Learning to manage fatigue requires changes in the way you think about yourself, changes in the way you do tasks, changes in your routines and habits, and involves help from your family and friends.

This book will work best if you read the chapters in order and if you do the exercises and activities throughout. There is no magic pill for managing fatigue, and this book does not suggest that you stop taking medication that your doctor has prescribed. However by learning the techniques in this book, in addition to any medication you are taking, you should begin to feel more in control of your life and your symptoms of fatigue.

Additionally, managing your fatigue should not be something you try and do alone. By involving loved ones, friends, co-workers and health care professionals, you will have a greater chance of being successful. It may seem that you are "giving in" to your multiple sclerosis if you ask someone else to cook dinner, or drive the kids to activities, however, if you are then able to enjoy more quality evening time helping with homework or reading at bedtime, isn't the payoff worth asking for the help?

You will need to take an honest look at your priorities, to not attach who you are to what you can or cannot do. It is also important to understand that change takes time and patience. Be kind to yourself, applaud your successes and don't get down on yourself if you can't stick to your new behaviors 100% of the time. It takes around 6 months to develop a new habit. Learn to laugh at your mistakes, tell others what you are trying to do so they can help you.

If you are feeling the need for more formal support and instruction, there are professionals who are available as well. An occupational therapist can teach you many of the energy management techniques in this book. They can also look at your environments and make suggestions for ways to make these work better, they can also show you adaptive equipment that might be useful. A physical therapist can help you develop an exercise routine and talk to you about external supports for walking, such as a cane, walker, or scooter. A psychologist or social worker can help you with anxiety or depression, two conditions that may impact how tired you feel. In addition there are professionals who can help you with clutter, housekeeping, exercise and even doing errands.

I hope that this book provides you with ideas to help you feel more empowered and better able to manage your fatigue. The techniques in this book may also be helpful for those without multiple sclerosis. If you know others who are trying to fit everything in to busy lives, teach them the techniques that you learn throughout this book.

Nancy Lowenstein, MS, CTR, BCPR

ACKNOWLEDGMENTS

I want to thank all the individuals with multiple sclerosis who have taught me so much over the years about how MS affects them on a daily basis. Also my colleagues at the Mount Auburn Hospital Comprehensive Multiple Sclerosis Care Center for their support of this project, especially Ann Pisani, RPT for her help with the chapter on exercise. Last, but not least all my occupational therapy students who volunteered to assist with this project, some who wrote whole chapters and others, like Allyson Marvin, who provided outlines.

FIGHTING FATIGUE IN MULTIPLE SCLEROSIS

1

Busy Lives, Busy Minds, and Busy Bodies

Nancy Lowenstein, OTR

Conserving your energy was probably not something you thought about before you were diagnosed with multiple sclerosis. You were able to go through your day without worrying about when you were going to "hit the wall." You managed all aspects of your life, from personal needs to family demands to work and leisure time. Now, however, you find yourself losing energy by midmorning or later. The tank gets empty much quicker and is harder to refill. By the end of the day, you are wondering, "What did I do today that made me so tired?" This chapter will help you to realize that your daily life is very energy consuming, even if you don't think so. Throughout this book, you will learn about your daily activities and which ones take a lot of your energy and which ones help to restore your energy.

> **In this chapter you will learn**
> - The importance of habits and routines
> - Where your energy may be leaking out
> - How emotions and stress impact your energy levels

Night Owl or Lark?

Our energy levels naturally ebb and flow in cycles throughout the day. These are called circadian rhythms. We each have our own patterns and preferences: some of us are "morning" people; others are "night owls." Some people jump right out of bed, ready to attack the day, and others take awhile to hit their stride. Take the quiz, "Are You a Night Owl?" to see if you are a night owl, a morning person, or an intermediate.

Maybe you are a night owl who has learned to live in a morning world. You may still have these natural patterns and, with multiple sclerosis, your old patterns may be taking over again. Learning about your daily patterns and how to manage your day in accordance with your natural energy cycles is an important aspect of managing fatigue.

Why am I so tired if I haven't done anything yet?

For as long as you can remember, you've performed many daily tasks. It's gotten to the point that, now, you don't even think about them anymore. These are called habits and routines. Habits are those activities that you do automatically,

QUIZ

Are you a Night Owl?

Think about a time before you had multiple sclerosis when answering these questions.

In the morning,

1. I don't usually rely on an alarm clock or I wake and get out of bed as soon as the alarm rings.
2. I hit the snooze button. I hit the snooze button. I hit the snooze button. Eventually, I drag myself out of bed.

At 9:30 in the evening,

1. I have been in bed for an hour.
2. I am doing the laundry, vacuuming, and baking bread.

The time of day that I am most alert and energetic is

1. Early morning.
2. Afternoon.
3. Late evening.

If you answered 2, 2, 3, you are a night owl; if you answered 1, 1, 1, you are an early bird. An intermediate person may respond to some questions as a night owl and to others as an early bird; intermediates are often able to be more flexible with their schedules. This information was originally published in *Birds of a Different Feather* by Carolyn Schur and is used with permission of the author and Schur-Goode Associates.

without thinking. When performing habits, you can multi-task. For example, you can usually get dressed while talking on the phone or checking email, without forgetting what you're doing (except if you have cognitive problems—problems with thinking or memory). When you get into your own car, you don't think about where your key goes; you simply put the key in the ignition. Routines are a series of tasks, such as a child's bedtime routine or a morning routine, which may consist of showering, dressing, and getting coffee.

The habits and routines that you have performed without thinking for so many years can now seem exhausting, and you may wonder why. For one thing, many of these activities consume high levels of energy. Showering is akin to aerobic activity. In the shower, you stand, bend, reach, and move your arms and legs nonstop for 15 to 20 minutes. Then, you get out of the shower and dry yourself, which involves more standing, bending, and reaching. Then, you get dressed, during which you stand, bend, and reach some more. Finally, you make breakfast, which involves even more standing, bending, and reaching! Of course you're tired—you just had an aerobic workout! If you have balance problems, spasticity, or pain, you have been working even harder—expending even more energy. And this is only your morning routine. What if you are a parent caring for young children who need you to bathe, dress, and feed them, or what if you need to drive 40 minutes in stressful rush-hour traffic?

I think by now you get the point that your daily activities involve a lot more than you may realize and that, when you string together a series of routines, you may simply be burning through all of your energy and all of your reserves.

To understand how you spend your time and where your energy might be going, it may be helpful for you to list the routines and habits that you engage in on a regular basis. Use Chart 1 to list your routines and then list the "habits" or activities that make up each routine.

I don't want to give in to my multiple sclerosis, so I need to walk a lot

Multiple sclerosis causes multiple physical symptoms—muscle weakness, spasticity, difficulty walking, tremors, ataxia, and pain, to mention a few. If you have any of these symptoms, you'll need to expend more effort to move correctly or to maintain proper posture. Fighting these physical symptoms by walking without the support of assistive devices, such as a cane, rollator, walker, or leg orthotics, is a huge source of lost energy. Your body is working extra hard to move correctly, and you will fatigue more quickly just by trying to compensate for your physical issues. It is important to consider these issues as you look at managing your fatigue. Perhaps you'll want to use a device to help you manage your physical symptoms, in the same way that you may be taking medications to manage other symptoms. In Chart 2, list your physical symptoms, how they affect you, and what you might be able to do about them.

I sit at a desk all day, why do I feel tired?

You've now looked at your routines, habits, and physical symptoms, but other activities that you may not have considered may be causing your fatigue. We all know that being physically active can make us tired, but using "cognitive"

Chart 1

Habits and activities that make up my daily routine

Routine	Habits/activities
Morning routine (example)	Shower Groom (make-up, shave, dry/style hair) Dress Make a light breakfast

_____

_____

_____

_____

_____

_____

_____

_____

_____

_____

_____

_____

_____

_____

_____

Chart 2

Physical symptoms: How they affect me and what I can do about them

Physical symptoms	How it affects me	What I can do about it

energy, that is using our minds, can result in fatigue as well.

Reflect on a time when you had to sit in a class, meeting, or other venue in which you were listening and thinking more than you were moving around. Were you tired at certain times? Did you look at your watch to see when the event would be over? Did you leave at the end of the class or meeting feeling exhausted? Just like your body, your mind requires energy to run. Being in a meeting or classroom requires you to sit still but upright, to process what many people are saying, and to remain focused on multiple sources of input, perhaps a document, a presentation, and a speaker all at once. Even if you don't have any cognitive impairment, your mind must work very hard to manage all of these inputs. If you do have cognitive impairments, you will use even more cognitive energy in these situations. Take some time to think about all of the cognitive tasks that you complete on a daily basis—these include cognitive tasks both at work and at home—and write down your tasks in Chart 3.

Have you ever noticed that you feel tired even after doing an activity while sitting down, such as crafts, computer work, or even preparing a meal? Why is sitting down and not doing anything physical so tiring? The answer lies in the mechanics of muscles: when you are sitting, you are asking your trunk muscles to support your body in an upright fixed position for long periods of time; your arms are being held in a fixed, and perhaps, unsupported position (see ergonomics in Chapter 7); and your head is also being held in a flexed forward and fixed position. These fixed positions require your muscles to hold contractions for long periods of time to keep you in the positions, and, by not moving around, you are not increasing your blood

Chart 3

Cognitive tasks that I regularly do at home and at work

I regularly do the following cognitive tasks

_____

_____

_____

_____

_____

_____

_____

_____

_____

_____

_____

_____

_____

_____

_____

_____

_____

flow. Additionally, your eyes are working very hard to remain focused on the task. Include the mental activity of attending to the task, and it all adds up to very large energy consumption. This holds true whether you are doing the task for leisure, fun, or work.

Reflect on the amount of time that you spend each day on tasks while you are seated. You can use the examples in Chart 4 to get started.

Chart 4

Time spent on various sedentary activities

I sit in one place for _____ minutes at a time when doing a task.

I look at the computer screen for _____ minutes without a break.

I sit in or drive a car for _____ minutes without a stretch break.

Emotional energy

Our emotions also eat up valuable energy. Anger, depression, and stress all require large amounts of "emotional" energy. A variety of biologic processes take place when your emotions are high. During stressful times, your body produces chemicals to help you cope with the situation. These substances increase blood flow, reaction time, and the rate of other biologic process. When the stressor is removed, your body goes into a relaxed state again, leaving you more tired than before you were stressed. Long-term stress can have an impact on your health and immune system as well, so it is important to be realistic when looking at your own stress levels and to seek help from an appropriate professional. It is not possible to avoid everyday tensions, but it is important to recognize the role that stress plays in fatigue and to learn how to manage stress. Think about areas in which you expend emotional energy, and jot your thoughts down in Chart 5.

Chapter Summary

In this chapter, you learned that your daily energy is finite and that there are many ways that the steam seeps out of you throughout the day. You may not even be conscious of the many ways that you lose energy. Your daily routines and habits, your cognitive tasks, and your emotions all require energy. Whether you are a day or night person will be an important factor when it comes to figuring out how to create a more efficient routine. This book will help you to explore all of these areas and to learn skills that may help prevent your strength from "leaking" out during the day.

In the next chapter, you will take a look at how your days are structured and examine how this structure may be having an impact on your fatigue levels.

Reference

Night Owl Network. Are you a night owl? Available at http://www.nightowlnet.com/archive06.htm. Accessed on October 7, 2008.

Chart 5
How I expend emotional energy

Things that regularly stress me	I get angry easily when	I feel depressed and sad about
_____		
_____		
_____		
_____		
_____		
_____		
_____		
_____		
_____		
_____		
_____		
_____		
_____		
_____		

2

A Look at Your Daily Routine

Nancy Lowenstein, OTR

An important part of learning how to manage your fatigue is looking at what you do during a typical day. Energy can just leak, out and you are left wondering, "What did I do today, and why am I so tired?" It is important to remember that all activities use energy. Understanding how much energy each activity uses and having ways to renew your energy throughout the day will help you to better manage your fatigue.

In this chapter you will learn
- About habits that can be problematic
- How to categorize your daily routines and habits
- How to create a daily activity log to analyze

Habits that can cause problems

The habits and routines that you have had for a lifetime may be difficult to change. Additionally, who you are is often embedded in what you can do or accomplish. You may have always had an excellent memory for names, or maybe your claim to fame was that you could go all day on a cup of coffee and a muffin. However, now that you have multiple sclerosis, your memory may not be as good and you may forget names, or you may be tired after simply taking a shower, and the cup of coffee doesn't help rev up the engines anymore. These changes in your self-perception may be difficult to accept. You may resist making the necessary changes to manage your multiple sclerosis and energy needs because these changes also alter your self-perception. Embracing the changes and learning how to take control of your symptoms of multiple sclerosis can empower you. Making these changes doesn't mean that you have to give up the activities that you like; instead, you may need to learn new ways to do these activities, arrange your schedule, and maybe even ask others for support. For others, making a few key changes in their daily routines may be all that they need to keep their engines running during the day. Even so, making adjustments can be difficult.

Habits that can cause problems
- Being too independent; not asking for help
- Being too spontaneous; not wanting to plan ahead
- Juggling too many things at once
- Wanting to "do it all"

A typical day

Typically, you engage in a variety of different activities during the day. Table 1 provides an example of a completed activity chart for a single day. You have to do some of these activities yourself—no one else can do them for you; others have to be done, but you might be able to delegate them to someone else. You may have still other activities that you

Table 1: Typical daily activities

Activities that you have to do	Shower, dress, eat
Activities that can be delegated	Grocery shopping, laundry, cooking, cleaning, etc.
Activities that could be restructured	Work, childcare, exercise, etc.
Pleasurable activities	Hobbies, movies, socializing

have to perform, but you might be able to structure them differently so that you use less energy, and, finally, you have some activities that you enjoy, that you find pleasure in performing. However, these pleasurable activities are often the ones that you give up first, when, in fact, these activities may also be activities that will help rejuvenate or restore your depleted energy. Now it's your turn to write down your daily activities—where would you put them (Activity 1)?

You may also believe that, when you perform an activity while sitting down, you may not be expending a lot of energy. However, simply sitting down doesn't make an activity relaxing or rejuvenating. Working on a computer is

Activity 1 Typical daily activities

Activities that you have to do

_____

_____

_____

_____

_____

Activities that can be delegated

_____

_____

_____

_____

_____

Activities that could be restructured

_____

_____

_____

_____

_____

Pleasurable activities

_____

_____

_____

_____

_____

an activity that is often thought of as relaxing, but it actually takes a lot of energy to work on a computer: your eyes are focused, your mind is very busy processing the information on the screen, and your muscles are working to keep your body correctly positioned. This is not relaxing! Sitting down and concentrating on a task—whether it be a hobby, work activity, or paying bills—also uses a lot of mental and physical energy, making the task more tiring than you think.

Where does my energy go?

To understand how you use your energy, it is important to identify your personal activity profile. This is a way of looking at how different activities may affect your fatigue levels, that is, how much an activity tires or rejuvenates you. You often don't realize how much energy an activity takes because, previously, you hadn't had to think about it.

If you are interested in creating your activity profile to understand how you may manage your fatigue, here is an exercise to help get you started. You can use the form at the end of this chapter to make photocopies, as it is best to track your activities over several days, including a weekend day and a weekday. You can also make up your own format that you personalize for your needs.

Creating your activity profile

The chart at the end of this chapter is divided into several columns. These are time, activity, fatigue level, symptoms, and comments.

For each hour during the day, briefly note the activity or activities that you have been doing. In the fatigue column, note, on a scale of 1 to 10, how tired you feel during or after doing the activity (1= not at all tired to 10 = exhausted) or note with an *R* any activity that felt relaxing and restored your energy. In the column marked *Activity Priority*, write down a number between 1 and 5. Table 2 provides the definitions of these numbers.

Take a moment to write down your activities from a typical weekday and weekend day on a sheet of paper, start from the time you wake up, and stop when you go to sleep. Don't skip anything, and ask someone to help you if you can't remember your activities.

Table 2: Scoring guide for activity priorities

1 = Activity has to be done by me, and it works fine the way it is (e.g., getting dressed)
2 = Activity has to be done, and it could be delegated to someone else (e.g., grocery shopping)
3 = Activity has to be done by me, but I need to look at how to change the activity so it isn't so tiring (e.g., work, taking a shower)
4 = Activity that I like doing and don't want to give up (e.g., going out with friends)
5 = Activity that doesn't have to be done; it's a bonus if I have enough energy (e.g., cleaning the closets)

In the symptom column, note any symptoms you feel during or after doing the activity (e.g., blurred vision or stiff muscles), and, finally, in the comment column, note anything else about this activity that you feel is important. See the example of a completed Activity Profile in Table 3. Alternatives to trying to remember all of your activities when completing an activity log, but still obtaining this important information, could be to look at your planner for the way you spend your days.

Rate and rank your daily activities

Now that you have completed your activity logs, it's time to figure out what it all means. When you're battling fatigue, it's common to get rid of your fun activities and fill up your days with the "have to dos" or important activities before you run out of energy. This creates an imbalance in your life by focusing too much on the mundane and necessary activities and not creating time for fun or restorative activities. Leisure activities can help to alleviate stress and even fatigue, especially while you're engaged in the activity. When you're doing something you enjoy, your brain creates dopamine, a chemical that enhances your pleasure centers and gives you a feeling of well-being. Your focus is on the activity because it is enjoyable, and you will not feel tired.

Analyzing your activity log and setting daily priorities

You will now want to look at your activity logs to try to identify patterns around your fatigue. You can look for patterns in many different ways. Patterns can be related to the time of day; for instance, you may not feel fatigued until a certain time of the day. Patterns may be related to symptoms; some people with multiple sclerosis develop blurred vision before they become fatigued. Patterns may be related to activities; for example, doing a certain activity may increase your fatigue level. Finally, patterns may be related to activities that are not fatiguing but, instead, are

Table 3: Example of a completed 24-hour activity profile

Time	Activity	Fatigue level
5:00 AM		
6:00	Wake at 6:30	3
7:00	Wake son; shower self	8
8:00	Drive son to school; walk dog	10
9:00	Eat breakfast; read paper	4
10:00	Start laundry	6
11:00	Computer Internet, email, games	2
12:00 PM	Computer Internet, email, games	8
1:00	Pick up son at school; take him to the dentist	10
2:00	Take son to music lesson	10
3:00	Grocery shopping	10
4:00	Home; walk the dog	10
5:00	Make dinner	10
6:00	Dinner	8
7:00	Clean up; watch TV	8
8:00	Bedtime reading to son	R
9:00	Bed	R
10:00	Sleep	
11:00	Sleep	
12:00AM	Woke to go to bathroom	

Activity priority	Symptoms	Comments
N/A	Morning stiffness	
1		Use a tub seat for shower
2; 4	Legs wobbly	
1		Felt less tired after sitting
2		Up and down stairs
4		
4	Blurred vision, headache	Forgot to eat lunch
1	Headache, urinary frequency, stiffness	
1	Same	
1		Lights bothered my eyes
2	Legs very stiff	
1	Headache, forgetful	
1		
2		
3	Muscles very tired	Fell asleep on son's bed; husband woke me to go to our bed
N/A		

rejuvenating—those that give you energy. Once you have found patterns, you can try and find solutions.

Use the charts provided in Tables 4 and 5 to analyze your activity logs and look for patterns.

You have now taken a look at how your day is structured, what makes you most tired, what rejuvenates you, what symptoms to be aware of, and how you build your day with necessary, fun, or other tasks. This is the foundation from which to build your energy management skills.

Table 4: Activities: Fatigue related to various activities and priority ratings

	How tired does this make you (1–10)	Activity priority#
Activities I have to do		
Activities I can delegate		
Activities I can restructure		
Activities I like to do		

Summary

In this chapter, you looked at your habits and routines and a typical day more closely to identify patterns that may contribute to your feelings of fatigue or of increased energy. Additionally, you looked at which activities you might be able to delegate, change, or add to your daily routine. In the next chapter, you will use this information to decide how to make changes in your daily routines to manage your fatigue.

Table 5: Activities
Identify how many of each numbered activity you had during each day that you kept an activity journal

Day	1	2	3	4
1 = Activity has to be done by me				
2 = Activity has to be done, and I could delegate to someone else				
3 = Activity has to be done by me. I need to look at how to change the activity so it isn't so tiring				
4 = Activity that I like doing and don't want to give up; my fun activities				
5 = Activity that doesn't have to be done; it's a bonus activity that I can do if I have enough energy				
FATIGUE LEVEL				
Activities that make me most fatigued were (over 8 on the fatigue scale) **Day**	1	2	3	4

Continued on next page

Table 5: Activities, *continued*

FATIGUE LEVEL, *continued*				
Activities that make me somewhat fatigued were (between 4 & 7 on the fatigue scale) **Day**	1	2	3	4
Activities that make me least fatigued were (2–3 on the fatigue scale) **Day**	1	2	3	4
Activities that restored my energy **Day**	1	2	3	4

Table 5: Activities, *continued*

SYMPTOMS					
I noticed the following symptom(s) when I was getting fatigued or already fatigued **Day**	**1**	**2**	**3**	**4**	
PATTERNS					
I noticed the following patterns regarding my fatigue, symptoms, or activities **Day**	**1**	**2**	**3**	**4**	

My Activity Profile

Use this chart to create your own activity profile. Make copies of it and fill this out for a few days, make one a weekend day and one or two weekdays. Use the following scales for each section:

Fatigue: 1= not at all tired to 10 = exhausted; R=relaxing/rejuvenating

Activity Priority:

1 = Activity has to be done by me, and it works fine the way it is (e.g., getting dressed)

2 = Activity has to be done, and I could delegate to someone else (e.g., grocery shopping)

3 = Activity has to be done by me; I need to look at how to change the activity so it isn't so tiring (e.g., work, taking a shower)

4 = Activity that I like doing and don't want to give up (e.g., going out with friends)

5 = Activity that doesn't have to be done; it's a bonus activity that I can do if I have enough energy (e.g., cleaning the closets)

Time	Activity	Fatigue level	Activity priority	Symptoms	Comments
5:00AM					
6:00AM					

My Activity Profile, *continued*

Time	Activity	Fatigue level	Activity priority	Symptoms	Comments
7:00AM					
8:00AM					
9:00AM					
10:00AM					

Continued on next page

My Activity Profile, *continued*

Time	Activity	Fatigue level	Activity priority	Symptoms	Comments
11:00AM					
12:00PM					
1:00PM					
2:00PM					

Continued on next page

My Activity Profile, *continued*

Time	Activity	Fatigue level	Activity priority	Symptoms	Comments
3:00PM					
4:00PM					
5:00PM					
6:00PM					

Continued on next page

My Activity Profile, *continued*

Time	Activity	Fatigue level	Activity priority	Symptoms	Comments
7:00PM					
8:00PM					
9:00PM					
10:00PM					

Continued on next page

My Activity Profile, *continued*

Time	Activity	Fatigue level	Activity priority	Symptoms	Comments
11:00PM					
12:00AM					

3

It's All so Important!
What Can I Change?

Nancy Lowenstein, OTR, and
Nadia D'Arista, OTS

In this chapter, you will learn how to look at your activities, tasks, routines, and habits and decide which to keep, change, or delegate. How do you change your routines and habits to make them more efficient and to expend less energy? You can modify an activity in many ways; you may need to experiment with different methods before you find the best way for you. Think about three areas when you are trying to change an activity: (1) Do you need to change yourself?, (2) Do you need to change how the activity is done?, or (3) Do you need to change the environment in which the activity takes place? Let's use the example of taking a shower: changing yourself may lead you to exercise your quadriceps so that you can lift your leg over the edge of the tub; changing the activity may mean taking a shower at night instead of in the morning; changing the environment may mean using a tub seat or even taking a shower in a different bathroom in the house.

In this chapter you will learn how to modify or adapt your daily tasks or routines by
- Changing something about yourself
- Changing something about the activity
- Changing something about the environment

Changing something about yourself

Each person with multiple sclerosis will have a unique experience. Additionally, multiple sclerosis causes many different symptoms, and the symptoms can vary from day to day. One day, you may be very stiff; another day, you may be able to move more comfortably. Changing yourself may be difficult, but you can begin by simply thinking about what you need or want to change. You may want to incorporate exercise into your daily routine or learn yoga or meditation. Perhaps you want to change the day or time that you take your medication (after checking with your physician), or you may even want to try a medication that you have not ever taken. Maybe your biggest change may simply be trying to get more sleep.

In the exercise shown in Table 1, you will use the information that you identified in your activity log in Chapter 2. List here those activities that you rated above a 6 on the fatigue scale, and see if there is something that you can change about yourself to make the activity less tiring.

Table 1: Activities that I participate in on a regular basis: What can I change about myself to make the activity consume less energy?

Activity	Change in Me

When should you perform activities?

When you analyzed your activity log, you identified patterns to your fatigue; these may have included being more tired in the afternoon or, conversely, waking up tired and getting more energy by noon. As we discussed in Chapter 1, you may be more of a morning person or you may be a night person. Your energy level will vary throughout the day. Your mood may be different, and performing a task may be less difficult at certain times. Also, some activities, such as exercising and eating healthy snacks, can increase your energy levels. Whatever your particular pattern, complete the most energy-consuming activities during the part of the day when you feel the most energized. Later chapters in this book will discuss how to balance your daily, weekly, and monthly routines. Use Table 2 to look at the time of day that you complete your high-energy activities.

Table 2: High-energy activities and performance times

Activities that take take a lot of energy	Usually performed at this time	Try to perform at this time

Change something about the activity

Making significant modifications to the tasks themselves will have the biggest impact your fatigue level. You can make these changes in a variety of ways, and, as you think about your different routines, habits, and activities, you may even see that you've already made changes to some of them without even realizing it. In this section, you will learn ways to make changes to the number of steps, sequence of steps, time of day, or amount of time it takes to complete an activity. You will also learn to make changes to the tools, equipment, or materials that you use to perform the activity, breaking the task into smaller chunks, and varying who completes the activity or asking someone to help you with all or part of the activity. Let's look at each of these different ways to modify an activity. To do this, we will look at a task that has lots of steps, such as baking cookies from scratch, and use this example for all the methods so that you can get an idea of the many ways of changing the same activity.

Change the sequence or number of steps

To figure out how to alter the sequence of the steps or to eliminate steps in any activity, you first have to list the key steps of the task. Now let's look at this list of the key steps in baking cookies from scratch (Table 3) and see how you can do this in fewer steps (Tables 4).

By first gathering all of the ingredients, measuring tools, and other equipment at once and putting them all on the workspace, you are able to reduce the number of steps and save energy by not walking, bending, and reaching more than is necessary. You may even be able to think of other ways to save steps.

Change the time of day or amount of time needed to do an activity

When making cookies, you can choose when to bake them: during the hottest time of day, with the oven then adding heat to an already-hot kitchen, or later in the day or early in the morning. You can also make them during the time of day when you have the most energy. You could use a quicker method, such as using a commercial mix or a slice-and-bake cookie dough. You can premix all of the dry ingredients, keeping the mix in a container, so that you

Table 3: Steps involved in baking cookies from scratch

1. Take out or find the recipe

2. Preheat the oven

3. Take out the mixer

4. Take out and grease a cookie sheet

5. Take out the butter, put it into a bowl, and beat

6. Take out and measure the sugar

7. Add the sugar to the bowl with the butter and beat

8. Take out the eggs, add them to the butter and sugar mixture, and beat

9. Take out and measure the vanilla; add it to the butter, sugar, and egg mixture; and beat

10. Take out and measure the flour

11. Take out and measure the baking powder and salt

12. Add all of the dry ingredients to a bowl and mix

13. Add the dry ingredients to the butter, sugar, egg, and vanilla mixture and mix together

14. Spoon individual cookies onto a cookie sheet

15. Put the cookie sheet into the oven, and set the timer

16. Remove the cookie sheet from oven, remove the cookies from the sheet, and place the cookies on a cooling rack

17. Place the cooled cookies into a container

18. Clean up

Table 4: Steps involved in baking cookies from scratch (modified)

1. Take out the recipe

2. Preheat the oven

3. Take out the mixer, measuring cups and spoons, and cookie sheet, and place all of the items on the workspace

4. Gather all of the ingredients and place them on the workspace

5. Combine all of the dry ingredients

6. Beat the butter and sugar together

7. Add the eggs and flavoring to the butter and sugar mixture

8. Add the dry ingredients to the mixture and beat together

9. Spoon the cookies onto a nonstick cookie sheet

10. Put the cookie sheet into the oven and set the timer

11. Remove the cookie sheet from the oven, remove the cookies from the sheet, and place the cookies on a cooling rack

12. Place the cooled cookies into a container

13. Clean up

only have to cream together the wet ingredients and then add the dry ones when you're in the mood for fresh-baked cookies. If you always bake holiday cookies, but you get tired because of all the other obligations you have, you might want to bake your cookies early, before the mad rush, and then freeze them. Many cookies can be frozen with good results.

Change the materials, tools, or equipment

Before we begin this discussion, let's define a few terms.

- **Materials:** Materials can be anything that is disposable or used only once. Examples include flour, butter, or eggs.
- **Tools:** Tools are things that you need to use to complete the activity; they are usually items that you can hold in your hand. Examples include measuring cups and spoons, spatulas, or a cookie sheet.
- **Equipment:** Equipment includes those items that are larger and more mechanical than tools. Examples include a mixer, oven, or refrigerator.

Changing materials may be more difficult than changing the time of day in which you bake, for example, but using things like prechopped vegetables or different kinds of packaging may make changes in this area easier. The tools can be changed by size, weight, ergonomics, height, color, or various other ways. Lastly, equipment may need to be modified, moved to another place, or changed completely.

We can use the example of baking cookies to see how materials, tools, and equipment can be changed to decrease the amount of energy that you expend. In the realm of materials, you could change from a made-from-scratch batter to a commercially prepared cookie mix or slice-and-bake cookie dough. Tools that may be helpful include a nonstick cookie sheet or measuring cups and spoons that are lighter or have larger handles so your muscles don't have to work as much. Finally, a variety of equipment can be employed that requires less energy. Using a tabletop mixer instead of a handheld one will make it easier on your arms and use less of your energy. Baking your cookies in a wall oven instead of a stove top-oven combination will also be less tiring because you don't have to bend to put the cookies into and pull them out of the oven.

Break task into smaller chunks

Breaking a task into smaller chunks, may mean doing a part of the task, then resting and resuming the task later. When preparing cookies, one way to break the project into smaller chunks is to take out the ingredients and baking tools and then wait while the eggs and butter come to room temperature; another way is to prepare the dough, put it into the refrigerator, take a rest, and then return at a later time to bake the cookies.

Change who does the task or ask someone to help you

People with multiple sclerosis often have the expectation that, if they let go of doing something or ask for help to do it, then they are giving in to the disease. If you are of this mindset, then your way of thinking may be costing you lots of energy. Even if you give up doing a few things, you can still take care of your family in other ways, or, if you share the task with someone else, you can still enjoy social time. Certainly, if baking is something you enjoy doing, you may not want to ask someone else to bake the cookies, but, if you are baking simply because you always bake the holiday cookies and it is expected of you, then maybe this is a time to teach the art of baking holiday cookies to the next generation. In the same way, you could share the cookie baking with children, grandchildren, or other family members, letting them do a lot of the moving around, gathering of materials, etc, while you mix the batter. This can be a wonderful way to pass down family traditions and recipes, as well as a great time- and energy-saving technique. Lastly, think about whether you need to do the task, or can you ask someone else do it?

One caveat: when you ask other people to do a task, you have to let them do it their way!

I like to tell a story of when I had two small children and had to go down four flights of stairs and then to a different building to do our laundry. When my husband volunteered to take on the task, I had to let him do it his way; he didn't sort clothes, and everything went into the dryer. I quickly learned to buy cold-water detergent and keep any clothing I cared about out of the wash and do that myself. By making this change in my thinking, I was able to give up a very tiring task and use that time and energy for playing with my children, cooking dinner, or doing another task.

Now it's your turn to practice analyzing an activity or task using Table 5. Start with something easy, but it should be something that you do on a regular basis, so that you can easily list the key steps.

Change something about the environment where the activity takes place

The last area that you want to look at is where you usually do the activity. Ask yourself the following questions: Is this the only place to do it? Is the space set up in the most

Table 5: Changing the way you complete an activity

Activity/task steps	What steps can I eliminate?	What changes can I make to the sequence?	What changes can I make in the materials, tools, and equipment?	Where I can break it into smaller chunks?	Who can I get to do it?	With whom do I want to do it?

energy-efficient way? Is the equipment in this room the best for the task? Is the lighting appropriate for the task? What is the noise level in the space? Some activities have to take place in the space you do them, e.g., showering, laundry, grocery shopping. Other activities can be moved to a different space, e.g., you can move the computer to a room on the first floor so that you don't have to take the stairs every time you want to check your email. Chapter 7 will allow you to explore your environments in more detail, but keep in mind the impact that the space can have on the amount of energy that you are expending.

Summary

In this chapter, you looked at ways to change activities, tasks, habits, and routines to make them more energy efficient. Changing something about yourself, the activity, or the environment is key to doing this. By changing one of these, you may find a better way to perform the activity that is quicker or less tiring. Remember, when you try to change the way you do a task, it takes a while to feel comfortable with the new way of doing something. It may take practice, adjustments, and patience, but the payoff will be feeling less tired. In the next chapter, we will look at ways to restore your energy throughout the day.

4

Ways to Grab Some Rejuvenation

Daria Rabkin, OTS, and Nancy Lowenstein, OTR

W hen learning to manage fatigue, it is important to find ways to "fill the tank" throughout the day, preferably before you feel so tired that you can't recover. Rejuvenation is defined as something that "restores to a former state" or "makes you fresh or new again." Knowing what activities provide you with energy, or allow you to rejuvenate, is a key part of managing your fatigue. You will need to identify several activities that are rejuvenating because you will be in different situations and one method may not fit all of these situations. For some people, restoring energy can be accomplished by exercising, meditating, or eating right, but, for others, it may be more difficult to find restorative activities.

This chapter will speak to the various ways that an individual can decrease daily fatigue. Part of understanding how to manage your lack of energy is also understanding the signs your body is giving you that say, "Slow down!" Rather than ignoring these signs and plowing on, it is important that you respect these signs and use a restorative technique before your tank hits empty. Restorative techniques that will be discussed include getting enough sleep at night; taking naps or breaks during the day; using simple meditation, yoga, or T'ai- chi; eating right; finding leisure and enjoyable activities; exercising; and balancing your day.

In this chapter you will learn
- How to recognize the right restorative activities for you
- The importance of scheduling "down" or restorative time throughout your day

---

My energy bank

When you think of energy, it is helpful to have a visual image. You may find one of these two images helpful. Imagine a jar that holds your energy. When you wake in the morning, that jar is full, or nearly full; each time you do an activity, you either empty the jar or add to the jar. Some activities will consume and others will restore. In Chapter 2, you ranked how fatiguing or restorative you found different activities. You can go back to this exercise and, using the image of a jar, see how much energy you removed from the jar and how much you returned on your typical days. How did you come out at the end of the day? Did you have energy to spare or were you in the hole?

A second image that you can visualize is making deposits and withdrawals from a bank account. Every time you do an activity, you either remove or restore your own account. It is equally important for you to find ways to restore energy throughout the day. You will need to find activities that restore large or small amounts of energy and those that restore energy in a short period of time or require a longer period of time. This is so that you have choices throughout the day to restore your energy.

Getting enough sleep

Sleep is important for both physical and mental health, and getting enough sleep at night is essential for just about everyone. Eight hours is the most common recommendation, but an individual's need for sleep actually varies depending on several factors. These factors include

- Genetics
- The activities you do to control alertness (e.g., drinking coffee)
- The quality of your sleep
- Your unique sleep cycle
- The activities you do during the day (e.g., exercise)

All of these factors, plus your symptoms of multiple sclerosis, interact to determine how much sleep you may be getting. Though some of these factors, like genetics, cannot be controlled, it can be beneficial to adjust the ones that you can control if they are standing in the way of your getting a good night's sleep. Start with your neurologist; talk with him or her about your sleep and any symptoms (such as restless legs syndrome, bladder urgency or distention, pain, anxiety, or side effects from medications) that may be interfering with your sleep. Next look at your sleeping environment, i.e., your bedroom, and your sleep habits. Over the years, experts in sleep medicine have developed many helpful suggestions to improve sleep (Table 1).

Table 1: Tips to develop good sleep hygiene

- Set a fixed bedtime and wake-up time

- Make sure your bed and bedding are comfortable; old mattresses and pillows can be a major reason that you are not sleeping well

- Keep the room at a comfortable temperature and well ventilated

- Block out noise and light

- Do not use your bed as an office, TV, couch, etc.; it is for sleeping and intimacy only

- Develop a ritual to do before you go to bed; this might involve reading, drinking a warm glass of milk, or eating a banana

- Do NOT watch TV in bed; as a matter of fact, take the TV OUT of the bedroom

- If you can't go to sleep after 15–20 minutes, get out of bed, read, relax (no TV or computers), and then try again. (Do not try and convince yourself that you are ready to go to sleep)

The idea behind these suggestions is to make bedtime a habit with a consistent routine. Your brain will become aware of these cues and will begin to slow down when you start the routine. If you have children, you may remember creating a bedtime routine for them, such as singing a lullaby or reading a story to them. This routine served to help them calm down and be ready for sleep. As adults, we still need these bedtime routines. Take a moment and use Chart 1 to think about your current routine and how you can adapt it to create a bedtime routine that is more conducive to sleep.

Sleep deprivation has adverse effects on health (it can decrease the functioning of your immune system), alertness,

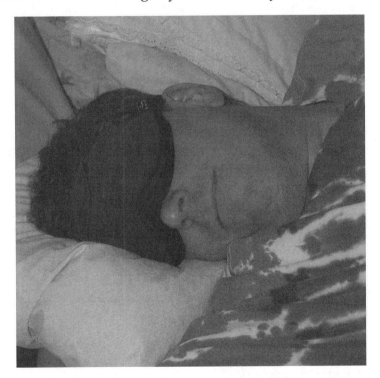

Image 1. Notice the eye mask and ear plugs to black out light and noise

Chart 1 Bedtime routines

Current routine	Y/N	Create a new bedtime routine
My bedtime is the same each night		
I get up at the same time each day		
I watch TV in my bed I read in bed		
My mattress is more than 6 years old My pillow is more than 6 years old		
My room is dark when I go to bed My room is quiet when I go to bed		
My room is a comfortable temperature for me, or I have enough bedding to make it comfortable		
I eat high-energy foods before I go to bed (sugary, caffeinated, alcohol)*		

*These foods should be avoided.

and performance and can, therefore, increase the amount of fatigue that you feel during the day. In other words, if you aren't getting enough sleep at night, you will be more tired, less focused, and less able to perform throughout the day.

Keeping a sleep diary, such as the one provided in Image 2, may help you figure out how fatigued or refreshed you are upon awakening, as well as what changes you may need to make during your day (e.g., taking a nap).

Sleeping

- An adequate amount of sleep is important for daily functioning
- Too little sleep has a negative effect on health, alertness, and performance
- Figure out what is causing your lack of sleep, and fix it!
- Talk with your doctor about your symptoms of multiple sclerosis and medications that may be affecting your sleep

---

Taking Naps

Another way to get some restoration during the day is to take a nap. When you have multiple sclerosis it is okay, and sometimes necessary, to nap. Several studies have concluded that humans are actually biologically prone to taking midafternoon naps. Have you ever wondered why toddlers and elderly people have a tendency to nap at that time? Well, now you know! The National Sleep Foundation encourages the use of naps to restore energy during the day and recommends various napping strategies.

National Sleep Foundation Sleep Diary

Fill out days 1-4 below and days 5-7 on page 2	COMPLETE IN MORNING						COMPLETE AT END OF DAY				
	I went to bed last night at:	I got out of bed this morning at:	Last night, I fell asleep in:	I woke up during the night: *(Record number of times)*	When I woke up for the day, I felt: *(Check one)*	Last night I slept a total of: *(Record number of hours)*	My sleep was disturbed by: *(List any mental, emotional, physical or environmental factors that affected your sleep e.g. stress, snoring, physical discomfort, temperature)*	I consumed caffeinated drinks in the: *(e.g. coffee, tea, cola)*	I exercised at least 20 minutes in the:	Approximately 2-3 hours before going to bed, I consumed:	Medication(s) I took during the day: *(List name of medication/drug(s))*	About 1 hour before going to sleep, I did the following activity: *(List activity: e.g. watch TV, work, read)*
DAY 1 DAY _____ DATE_____	_____PM/AM	_____PM/AM	_____Minutes	_____Times	☐ Refreshed ☐ Somewhat refreshed ☐ Fatigued	_____Hours		☐ Morning ☐ Afternoon ☐ Within several hours before going to bed ☐ Not applicable	☐ Morning ☐ Afternoon ☐ Within several hours before going to bed ☐ Not applicable	☐ Alcohol ☐ A heavy meal ☐ Not applicable		
DAY 2 DAY _____ DATE_____	_____PM/AM	_____PM/AM	_____Minutes	_____Times	☐ Refreshed ☐ Somewhat refreshed ☐ Fatigued	_____Hours		☐ Morning ☐ Afternoon ☐ Within several hours before going to bed ☐ Not applicable	☐ Morning ☐ Afternoon ☐ Within several hours before going to bed ☐ Not applicable	☐ Alcohol ☐ A heavy meal ☐ Not applicable		
DAY 3 DAY _____ DATE_____	_____PM/AM	_____PM/AM	_____Minutes	_____Times	☐ Refreshed ☐ Somewhat refreshed ☐ Fatigued	_____Hours		☐ Morning ☐ Afternoon ☐ Within several hours before going to bed ☐ Not applicable	☐ Morning ☐ Afternoon ☐ Within several hours before going to bed ☐ Not applicable	☐ Alcohol ☐ A heavy meal ☐ Not applicable		
DAY 4 DAY _____ DATE_____	_____PM/AM	_____PM/AM	_____Minutes	_____Times	☐ Refreshed ☐ Somewhat refreshed ☐ Fatigued	_____Hours		☐ Morning ☐ Afternoon ☐ Within several hours before going to bed ☐ Not applicable	☐ Morning ☐ Afternoon ☐ Within several hours before going to bed ☐ Not applicable	☐ Alcohol ☐ A heavy meal ☐ Not applicable		

Image 2. An example of a sleep diary. Reprinted with permission of the National Sleep Foundation, Washington, DC.

Benefits of Napping

- Increases alertness, energy, and productivity (especially if you did not get enough sleep the night before)
- Improves memory and the capacity for learning
- Improves health
- Increases relaxation
- Decreases stress

Taking a nap can help you to function better during the day. However, you should keep some important considerations in mind when it comes to taking a nap. These points will help you get the most out of your naps.

Special Considerations for Napping

- Try to nap either in the morning or just after lunch
- Decrease your consumption of caffeine and fatty food before napping
- Find a comfortable, clean, and darkened area to nap
- Grab a blanket and set your alarm (your cell phone likely has one)
- Do not rely on naps instead of getting a full night's sleep
- Keep your nap to one hour or less
- Take a nap when your children nap

Naps are meant to help rejuvenate you, but they will not be nearly as beneficial if you did not get enough sleep the night before.

Though naps can be incredibly helpful, they are not a substitute for a good night's sleep. It is also important to remember that taking a nap is not a sign of laziness—napping will help you become more productive, energetic, and alert for whatever the remainder of your day will bring.

Write down when and where you can take a nap during the day.

_____

_____

_____

_____

Taking breaks during the day

Similar to taking naps, taking breaks during the day will allow you to step away from whatever you may be doing and take a few minutes for yourself. Many people feel that they "have to do everything before I get tired" and are willing to work hours until they "hit the wall" and can go no further. Though this may get things done, it totally depletes your energy for the rest of that day and sometimes for the next day as well.

Taking breaks from doing activities that are tiring is very important. You can schedule a break from the task itself, or you can plan to follow a tiring activity with one that is more relaxing.

If you work at a computer or sit in the same position for more than an hour, it is important to schedule a 10-minute break to stretch, relax your eyes, and give your muscles a break. Taking breaks will give your body and mind a chance to replenish and will allow you to come back to your work or task at hand with a fresh set of eyes and a sharper focus. Figure out what helps you to restore your energy in a short period of time. Is it closing your eyes, listening to music, taking a walk? Try a few different things to see what works for you.

Taking Breaks
- Schedule a break approximately every hour
- Breaks will give your body and mind a chance to relax
- Breaks will allow you to come back to your work more refreshed and focused

---

Activities I want to try as a break from computer or other sedentary work

_____

_____

_____

_____

_____

_____

_____

_____

Yoga, T'ai-chi, meditation

Some people have found that activities such as T'ai-chi, yoga, or mediation are very helpful in teaching them ways to restore energy. Yoga and T'ai-chi have also been shown to have beneficial effects on balance and flexibility for individuals with multiple sclerosis. It is important to find an instructor who is familiar with multiple sclerosis or is open to helping you with any modifications that you might need. Meditation is a way of quieting your mind, slowing your heart rate, and providing a relaxed state of mind. As with learning any new skill, meditation takes practice and patience to learn, yet this is a great way to find rejuvenation any place, in a short amount of time.

Having a Good Diet

A good diet is balanced, including lots of different foods and not too much of any one food. This way, you get all of the nutrients that you need. Some foods (such as oily and fatty foods) can drag you down and decrease your energy, whereas other foods (like fruits and vegetables) can increase your energy, stamina, and focus.

Having breakfast will give you a boost of energy to start your day and may prevent you from feeling the need to overeat later in the day—which can lead to increased fatigue. An abundance of processed snacks and junk food will leave you with a bloated and dragging feeling because they are not filling; instead of eating processed foods, eat "real" food in moderation and savor it. Eating foods that provide wellness and power—such as vegetables, fruits (especially berries), whole grains, nuts and seeds (especially almonds and walnuts), organic dairy products, beans, and avocados—will also increase your energy and keep you from eating junk food. Additionally, you may need to monitor your intake of soda, caffeine, and sugary drinks because these beverages may give you a temporary bust of energy but leave you feeling tired later.

The National Multiple Sclerosis Society has several resources regarding nutrition and multiple sclerosis, including the nutrition tips to manage fatigue (Table 2).

Table 2: Tips to help manage fatigue

- Never go longer than four hours without food. You don't have to eat a lot. A small snack is fine.

- Shrink your meals so that you eat more frequently. For example, save half of your lunch, and eat it three hours later.

- Eat a small protein snack in the afternoon, such as a mozzarella stick, beef jerky, cottage cheese, or peanut butter, to help you feel more alert.

- Avoid big helpings. Avoid sugary desserts. Both will increase fatigue!

- Avoid over using caffeine. If you use caffeine as a pick-me-up throughout the day, it may lead to restless sleep and increased anxiety.

Eating Right
- Eat breakfast
- Eat more vegetables
- Eat real food in moderation; and savor it
- Eat wellness power foods, like nuts, grains and berries

Leisure activities and hobbies

When you have fatigue, it is often all you can do to meet your daily demands, so thinking about adding a leisure activity may seem like too much. However, doing things that give you pleasure is often rejuvenating. It may not be possible to continue your same leisure activity, such as running or knitting, so it is important to find something else that you can do to replace a cherished activity. People often substitute many hours of watching TV or sitting at the computer for their previous pleasurable leisure activities. Although watching TV and surfing the Internet can certainly give you pleasure, they do not occupy your mind in the same way that having a hobby or sharing an interest with someone else does. If you can't remember what you enjoyed doing in the past, or you are unable to do those activities because of your multiple sclerosis, use the space provided in Table 3 to brainstorm about other ideas for enjoyable activities and possible adaptations that you might need to do them. You might find it helpful to do this with a partner or someone else with whom you want to enjoy this play time. If you can't think of leisure activities that you used to enjoy, completing an interest checklist may be helpful to identify new activities (You can find a Modified Interest Check List at the end of this chapter).

But I am too tired to exercise!

Exercising regularly is important. Research has clearly documented that regular exercise is beneficial in combating fatigue for people with multiple sclerosis. You may feel that you are too tired to exercise, but, in the long run, exercise increases your capacity for activity. Exercise will help you get a better night's sleep and reduce your levels of

Table 3: Leisure activities old and new

Leisure activity that I love to do	Leisure activity that I want to try	Barriers	Adaptations I might need to make
Hiking	Bike riding	Poor balance	Use a bicycle built for two
Knitting	Knitting	Visual issues	Direct task lighting, large needles and bright colors

stress and anxiety. Doing some form of daily exercise is most beneficial because it is not the length of time, as much as it is the regularity of exercise, that matters. Consulting a physical therapist who is familiar with the unique needs of individuals with multiple sclerosis is important before you start any exercise program. (Chapter 5 provides more information about exercise and multiple sclerosis.) The key to using exercise as a rejuvenating activity is to remember that each day is going to be different, that doing a few minutes of exercise may be enough to get you going again, and that not overdoing exercise is important because too much exercise will make you more tired.

Creating a schedule for yourself will help you to remember the exercises that you should do during the day. Picking exercises that you can do sitting and standing will help you to easily incorporate them into your day. Try to do some kind of exercise every single day.

Exercising
- Pick exercises you enjoy doing
- Do at least 1-2 exercises a day
- Create an exercise schedule
- Spread out exercises throughout the day
- *Do not* overdo it!

Having a balanced life

It is important to know what goes into having a well-balanced life. While you are taking care of your kids, your home, and maybe your parents and working, where do *you*

Balance in Life
- Balance work, leisure, and sleep
- Prioritize activities that you have to do and those activities that you want to do

fit in? You have to fit in somewhere, and that's why it's important to have a healthy balance among all parts of your life. Balancing leisure time (doing activities that you enjoy and that will rejuvenate you, such as taking a walk or getting a massage or manicure) with work time (doing your job or something you find tedious) and with sleep time may be difficult—but it is nonetheless quite important. A balance in your life will help you prioritize and schedule activities that you have to do along with activities that you want to do (see Chapter 6 for more information on how to do this). Combining these areas equally creates a balance in your life that will allow you to feel happier, more energetic, and less fatigued.

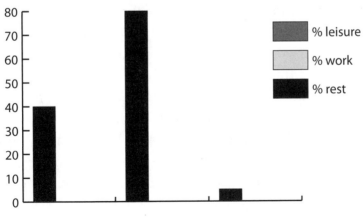

Image 3. A balanced day.

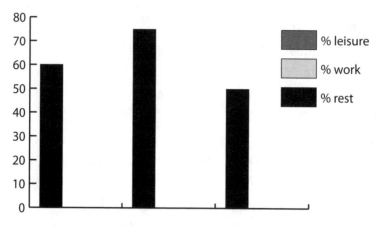

Image 4. An unbalanced day.

Summary

Being able to visualize your energy needs as either a jar that empties and refills or a bank account in which you make withdrawals and deposits may help you in thinking about where and when you need to make time for rejuvenation. When you are feeling fatigued, you can find ways to restore energy throughout your day or week. Getting enough sleep at night allows you to wake up refreshed and rejuvenated; taking naps and breaks during the day will help keep you focused on your task at hand when you return after your nap or break. Learning T'ai-chi, yoga, or mediation; finding a new hobby or leisure activity, or resuming a forgotten one; watching your diet and nutrition; and exercising regularly will all help increase your energy level. Finally, having a balance among work, leisure, and sleep will help you to manage your fatigue by allowing you to prioritize among the things that you have to do and the things that you want to do.

INTEREST CHECKLIST

| Activity | What has been your level of interest | | | | | | Do you currently participate in this activity? | | Would you like to pursue this in the future? | |
| | In the past ten years | | | In the past year | | | | | | |
	Strong	Some	No	Strong	Some	No	Yes	No	Yes	No
Gardening Yardwork										
Sewing/needle work										
Playing card										
Foreign languages										
Church activities										
Radio										
Walking										
Car repair										
Writing										
Dancing										
Golf										
Football										
Listening to popular music										
Puzzles										
Holiday Activities										
Pets/livestock										
Movies										
Listening to classical music										
Speeches/lectures										
Swimming										
Bowling										
Visiting										
Mending										
Checkers/Chess										
Barbecues										
Reading										
Traveling										
Parties										
Wrestling										
Housecleaning										
Model building										
Television										
Concerts										
Pottery										

Image 5. A Modified Interest Check List.

Resources and references

For more information and tips on sleep hygiene, check out the following websites:

- www.sleepfoundation.org
- www.stanford.edu/~dement/howto.html
- www.umm.edu/sleep/sleep_hyg.htm
- http://www.sleepeducation.com/Hygiene.aspx

Matsutsuyu J. The interest checklist. Am J Occup Ther 1969;23:323-8.

The University of Illinois at Chicago. The MOHO (Model of Human Occupation) Clearing House. Available at http://www.moho.uic.edu. Accessed on October 6, 2008.

National Multiple Sclerosis Society. You can ... maintain good nutrition. Available at http://www.nationalms society.org/living-with-multiple-sclerosis/you-can/main tain-good-nutrition/index.aspx. Accessed on October 6, 2008.

5

Incorporating Exercise into Your Daily Routine: the Importance of Exercise in Combating Fatigue

Sarah Hudak, MS, OTS, and
Nancy Lowenstein, OTR

Exercise has always been a key component in living a healthy lifestyle. Regardless of your age or sex, making time to incorporate exercise into your daily life can help you feel good and look good and can contribute to your overall health. Exercise can even help ease the symptoms of multiple sclerosis (MS). It can help you to retain your balance and flexibility, while regulating your sleep patterns, bowel movements, and appetite. Exercise can also help alleviate fatigue by building balance, flexibility, endurance, and strength so that you can perform your everyday activities. Today, however, going to gyms, joining yoga studios, and spending money on fitness gimmicks have been the primary ways that you think of for "working out." Incorporating strength into a daily routine is important, but, if you're wondering, "Do I have to go to the gym to have an exercise routine?" The answer is firmly, "No!" This chapter introduces ideas and strategies for incorporating exercise throughout your day, while highlighting the importance of exercise to sustain your well-being.

In this chapter you will learn
- The importance of exercise in combating fatigue
- Your supports and barriers to exercise
- Ways to incorporate exercise into your daily routine
- Different types of exercises that might be beneficial to you

---

Supports and barriers to exercise

Finding ways to condition your body or incorporating exercise into your daily routine can be challenging. For those who have never exercised or don't even like the thought of it, it's not as hard as you think! For those who enjoy exercising, but who now feel that exercising is more difficult because of MS and fatigue, it may be simply a matter of finding the right balance and learning to exercise within new limits. It is important to remember that, with MS, your daily abilities to exercise may vary. One day you may be able to take a 20-minute walk, and, the next day, 5 minutes may seem daunting. This variability should not cause you to skip exercising or to push yourself on a "bad" day; just understand that this is normal.

Barriers to exercise will be different for everyone. Some people can't find the time during the day, and others may have time but just don't know what activities to do. It is common for people with MS to be afraid to exert the energy necessary to exercise. They may think that their energy should be used elsewhere or fear not knowing what to do if something "bad" happens while exercising. The term "exercise" may haunt their thoughts! What are your fears? What barriers and supports do you have to exercise? You can use Table 1 to record some of your barriers and supports.

Common barriers to exercise

- Too tired: Don't have energy to spare!
- Unmotivated: Don't like it, don't want to try it, don't want to use it!
- Finances; Gym memberships are too expensive!
- Scared: What if something happens to me while I'm on a walk—Who's there to help?
- Difficulty getting to a gym, pool, or other facility

It is also important to understand what supports are available for you to exercise. For some people, it may be

---

Supports to exercise

- Paying for a club or gym membership
- Exercising with someone
- Being able to make exercise fun
- Having a specific exercise plan
- Not needing equipment
- Establishing a regular time to exercise everyday

---

paying for a gym or club membership; for others, it may be having someone with whom to exercise. Now, think about what supports you have for making exercise a regular part of your life, and record your supports in Table 1.

Table 1: My barriers and supports to exercise

My barriers	My supports

How will my diagnosis of MS affect my ability to exercise?

When you have MS and want to start an exercise program, it is best to start with an evaluation by a physical therapist who is familiar with the needs of individuals with MS. He or she can give you specific exercises for your particular needs. For instance, you may need to stretch or strengthen particular muscles, or you may need to work on balance. If you have spasticity, you may need to perform exercises in special ways. Common problem areas for those with MS are balance, strength, flexibility, and endurance. It is therefore very important to be able to figure out how to make sure that you do the exercises that are given to you on a regular basis.

What are the different types of exercise?

You may have heard of activities that work on strength, or balance, or endurance, but do you know what the differences are and why they are all important? MS affects the myelin sheath, the covering, around the nerves, which in turn affects the speed with which messages are sent from your brain to your muscles. If you have less myelin, your nerves are less efficient in sending messages, your muscles become weaker, and you may experience loss of strength, decreased range of motion in your major joints, and spasticity. Strength training can help prevent contractures (a permanent shortening of the muscles, which pulls the joint out of place), atrophy (a wasting away or shrinking of a muscle), and fatigue, while improving function. Exercises can be classified as resistive or nonresistive. Resistance can be accomplished by using weights, an exercise band, or even a one-pound bag of rice. Resistive exercises are used to increase muscle strength; by lifting against a resistance, you build muscle. You can slowly increase the amount of weight you use as you build muscle. When doing resistive exercises, it is important to not overdo it, as this can cause pain or muscle pulls. Nonresistive exercises are best for building up muscle endurance; endurance is how long you can move a muscle or hold it in a certain position. You need your muscles to be both strong and have good endurance.

Flexibility is another area that is important to address. Flexibility refers to how elastic your muscles and tendons are. Problems with flexibility can be caused by deconditioning, lack of activity, or spasticity. When you have decreased flexibility, you may have problems with walking, reaching, bending, or other activities. Exercises that address flexibility are also known as stretching. In this type of workout, it is important to hold the stretch for 20 to 30 seconds, relax, and then repeat the stretch, trying to go a little farther in the second stretch.

The last type of exercise is known as aerobic. Aerobic exercise works on cardiovascular fitness, which is important in combating fatigue. As your aerobic fitness improves, you will find yourself able to do more and have more energy. Aerobic activity is a low-intensity activity requiring high endurance over a continuous period of time. Riding a stationary bike, swimming in a pool, and going for a walk are all examples of aerobic activities. Difficulty with aerobic exercise can be a result of muscle weakness and limited endurance. If you choose to swim, it is important that the pool water temperature is between 80°F and 85°F. Ask what the normal temperature the pool is. If the pool in which you swim has an arthritis program, it will probably be too warm for someone with MS.

With any workout program, it is important to learn your limits. Starting small can help you understand what exercises work best for you.

How do I know what I need to incorporate into an exercise routine?

Discussing a routine with your physician, physical therapist, or occupational therapist is necessary before starting an exercise routine. Get as much information as possible, and ask questions! Exercise should be helpful, not hurtful. Before you go to a professional, you may want to ask yourself these questions to help guide your thinking.

- Do I need to work on my *balance*? Am I often falling over or having trouble sitting on my bed?
- Do I need to increase my *aerobic endurance*? Am I often tired after walking in the grocery store or while at work?
- How *flexible* am I? I know I'm not a gymnast, but can I comfortably bend and reach?
- Am I strong enough to do most of my daily tasks? Do I have enough strength to carry my child or lift shopping bags?

It is important to ask questions about yourself as well.

- What are my limitations? Do I know my limit? How do I know I've reached my limit?
- What are my goals for exercise? Do I want to be stronger? More balanced? More energized?
- What are my problematic symptoms?
- Do I know what I feel like when I am overtired?

Understanding potential risks to exercise: What should I do if I get overheated?

As an individual who wants to exercise, you should definitely understand your limits. If you don't know them, you could hurt yourself. Therefore, it is always important to be safe. Stretch before exercising. If using equipment, make sure that you know how to use it properly. Do you know where to find medical help, if needed?

Although many people sweat when exercising, overheating is an issue that people with MS are more likely to experience. Therefore, you may wish to employ a few techniques to prevent overheating while exercising and, if need be, to help cool off. Additionally, there are some important considerations to keep in mind as you plan your exercise program.

- Exercise in a cool room, place a fan near where you exercise, or exercise in an air-conditioned space
- Drink plenty of water before, during, and after exercise
- Exercise in a swimming pool with temperatures between 80°F and 85°F
- Wear light clothing made of a fabric, like cotton, that breathes
- "Precool" your body, and rinse your body with cool towels before beginning your exercise session
- To keep your body cool while you are exercising outside, use a cool towel or wrap behind your neck or wear a cooling vest
- Do not overdo it; listen to our body, and, if is telling you to stop, then stop

How to incorporate exercise into your daily routine

Media, gyms, and other social norms have told us that, for exercise to be useful, we need to spend a lot of time doing it. However, research has shown that exercise can be effective when done in smaller doses. The important part of any routine is to do it correctly, do it to your muscles' limits, and do it regularly. Some individuals like to set aside an hour to exercise; others find this too demanding. If the latter is you, there are ways to incorporate exercise into your daily routine so that exercise doesn't feel so demanding.

Table 2 includes some ideas on how to incorporate exercise into some very common daily activities.

Table 2: How to incorporate exercise into some very common daily activities

If you want to focus on...	...then use these "hidden" techniques
Balance	• Stand while brushing your teeth • Sit on a pillow while watching TV • Stand while you are waiting for a pot of water to boil or while something is toasting in the toaster
Aerobic endurance	• Walk while grocery shopping. If balance is a problem, push a cart for part of the trip • Go swimming • Park your car a few spots further away in parking lots • Be the one in charge of getting your newspaper at the end of the driveway
Flexibility	• If stretching on your bed, touch your toes and hold the stretch for 20 seconds while putting on your socks • During commercial breaks, stretch your back and legs • When you first wake up or during a time when you feel stressed out, use deep breathing to reach your arms to

continued on next page

Table 2: How to incorporate exercise into some very common daily activities, *continued*

If you want to focus on...	...then use these "hidden" techniques
Balance, *continued*	the ceiling and to your sides while stretching your back and arms • Take a break at work to stretch
Muscle strength	• While doing laundry, lift a heavy detergent container a few times • Take advantage of heavy food containers. • When doing dishes, hold onto the sink for support and do some squats

Summary

Regular exercise is important in helping you combat fatigue. It will help you overcome the complications from spasticity, muscle weakness, and decreased endurance from inactivity. A balanced exercise program will address strength, flexibility, balance, and cardiovascular health. It is important to consult with a healthcare professional who is familiar with the needs of people with MS, such as a physical therapist, before starting an exercise program. If you have MS, it is important for you to be careful to not overheat, to listen carefully to your body, to not overdo it, and to realize that, day-to-day, the type and amount of exercise that you can complete may vary. If you are not used to exercising, start slowly, and you will see benefits just by being active. If you are thinking about starting an exercise program, answer the questions in Table 3. You will discover your reasons for exercising and the roadblocks and support to getting started.

Table 3: Key questions to answer as you contemplate embarking on an exercise program

1. Is exercise important for me? ☐ Yes ☐ No
2. What are some reasons why exercise is important for people with multiple sclerosis?
_____
_____
3. What are some barriers that I will have to overcome in order to exercise?
_____
_____
3. What are some supports that I have to help me exercise?
_____
_____
4. What aspects of exercise can I incorporate into my routine?   Balance: ☐ Aerobic ☐ Endurance ☐ Flexibility ☐   Muscular Strength ☐ Other things I'd like to work on:
_____
_____
5. What do I need more information about before I can start exercise?
_____
_____

6

FITTING IT ALL IN

ANN WIGHTON, OTS, AND
NANCY LOWENSTEIN, OTR

"I'm so tired, but my son has to be picked up from hockey practice, my daughter's piano recital is tonight, the house is a mess, I have to go to the grocery store, and I have work piling up on my desk!" Sound familiar? Just thinking about it, is enough to make anyone feel exhausted. If you are a busy person, but also have multiple sclerosis-related fatigue, you may be wondering, "Is it even possible to fit it all in?" This chapter will help you look at your calendar from a larger perspective (daily, weekly, and monthly) and teach you how to create a balanced life that includes work, leisure, and restoration, while not running out of energy.

In this chapter you will learn how to

- Create organized weekly and monthly time schedules
- Assess how you are currently spending your time
- Reorganize your schedule to fit your priorities
- Adapt your schedule

Take the time to save time

When life gets busy, people have a tendency to stop planning and live "on the fly," just trying to keep up with life's demands. When you do this, you can miss valuable opportunities to save time and energy. The time and energy saved by good planning can dramatically lower your stress, another cause of fatigue! So, take a little time out of your day once a week to plan out a realistic daily schedule for yourself and then to review your plan. You will need a computer-based calendar program, a paper planner, an electronic device such as a PDA, a cell phone, or a plain old paper calendar. If you are responsible for other people's schedules, it may be good to purchase a large white board calendar to hang in a central place so that everyone can be involved in the scheduling and be aware of the demands on your schedule. You can use different colored markers for different people, appointments, social engagements, etc.

The weekly schedule

A weekly schedule is a 7-day schedule of tasks to be completed: appointments, social activities, meetings, exercise plans, etc. Remember that this schedule should be flexible and can be adjusted if higher-priority activities arise or your symptoms change. Don't forget to plan in rejuvenation or "me" time during each day as well.

A completed weekly schedule can paint a clear picture of which days have been overbooked and gives you enough time to reschedule events to ensure that the week is more balanced and manageable. The weekly schedule can help identify days that are less busy. Those less-busy days can be used to complete tasks of lower priority, or to participate in one-time high-energy activities (such as spreading mulch in your garden), because these activities should not to be coupled with other high-energy daily tasks. On the other hand, those less-busy days might be a good day to relax. Highly booked days may indicate a need to prioritize yours tasks (refer to Chapter 2) or may be an indicator that the previous day or following one should include more restorative time or fewer activities. Consider the energy level of each activity you schedule. If you have a very energy-consuming task to do on one day, make the other activities that day less energy consuming; for example, going out at night may mean rescheduling the grocery shopping to another day. Also look at how your hour-to-hour day is scheduled. If a task is very tiring for you, such as showering and dressing, then either split the tasks apart or follow them with a less energy-consuming task, such as eating breakfast.

To create your weekly schedule, either look at your daily log from Chapter 2 or write down your daily activities and note the ones that are very fatiguing and their priority (Chart 1). Using Chart 2, make a list of your daily activities and tasks, along with their fatigue and priority levels; you will use this list later in the chapter to create a weekly schedule.

Chart 1

Example of a daily activity log: fatigue level and activity priority

Time	Activity	Fatigue level	Activity priority
5:00 am			
6:00	Wake at 6:30	3	N/A
7:00	Wake son; shower self	8	1
8:00	Drive son to school; walk dog	10	2; 4
9:00	Eat breakfast; read paper	4	1
10:00	Start laundry	6	2
11:00	Computer internet, email, games	2	4
12:00 pm	Computer internet, email, games	8	4
1:00	Pick up son at school take to dentist	10	1
2:00	Son to music lesson	10	1
3:00	Grocery store	10	1
4:00	Home walk dog	10	2
5:00	Make dinner	10	1
6:00	Dinner	8	1
7:00	Clean up, watch TV	8	2
8:00	Bed	R	
9:00			
10:00			

Chart 2

Complete the daily activity log: fatigue level and activity priority

Time	Daily activity/ task/event	Fatigue level	Priority

The monthly schedule

A monthly schedule allows you to look at your schedule on a larger scale. It includes important events, appointments, and activities that may occur less frequently, such as a monthly book club or PTA meeting (Chart 3). Monthly schedules can guide you through your tasks week by week, thus making you feel more in control of your time and scheduling and thereby reducing fatigue. Looking at this schedule gives you an idea of which weeks may be partic-

Chart 3
Monthly activity log: frequency, fatigue level, and priority

Monthly activity/ task/event	Frequency of occurrence in a month	Fatigue level	Priority

ularly busy, allowing you the opportunity to reschedule events accordingly. For example, if the end of the month is heavily booked with important appointments and obligations, it may be wise to schedule your dinner party or evening out with friends for earlier in the month. Using Chart 3, write down those activities that occur regularly, but on a weekly, monthly or bimonthly basis, and note the fatigue level and priority for these, as you did in Chart 2.

GETTING STARTED: Create your own schedule

Blank templates of both weekly and monthly schedules are provided at the end of this chapter.

Weekly schedule: Plan the days of your week by entering tasks, activities, and events into the appropriate time slots (Chart 4). Keep in mind that you may experience daily patterns of symptoms or fatigue (refer to Chapter 2), and this should be considered when planning your weekly schedule. Under the column labeled "comments," comment on why tasks were not completed and how you felt overall that day (including your symptoms and fatigue). Keep these schedules so that you can analyze them later.

Monthly schedule: Enter important appointments and events, making sure to include activities that do not occur regularly each week. Use your monthly schedule as a guide when planning your weekly schedule (Chart 5).

Review how you are spending your time

Making a schedule—whether daily, monthly, or weekly—does not mean you can't change the schedule. If you have multiple sclerosis, you need to be flexible because, on any

Chart 4
Blank calendar to develop a weekly schedule

	SUN	MON	TUES	WED	THURS	FRI	SAT
5AM							
6AM							
7AM							
8AM							
9AM							
10AM							
11AM							
12PM							
1PM							
2PM							
3PM							
4PM							

Chart 4, *continued*

	SUN	MON	TUES	WED	THURS	FRI	SAT
5PM							
6PM							
7PM							
8PM							
9PM							
10PM							
11PM							
12AM							
1AM							
2AM							
Tasks not completed							
Comments							

Chart 5
Blank monthly calendar

SUN	MON	TUES	WED	THURS	FRI	SAT

given day, your fatigue may be too great for you to do what you had planned. When you have a weekly plan, however, you can look at that, see what is a high priority for that day, and make adjustments to the remainder of the week or month. To learn more about your patterns, you may find it helpful to review your weekly schedules at the end of each week and again after 3 to 4 weeks. Did you have days of the week or times of the day during which you were noticeably more fatigued? Was there a particular daily combination of activities that was difficult to accomplish together? Did you notice a successful combination of tasks and activities? Are there any patterns in your symptoms throughout the week related to your activities? What tasks didn't you accomplish and why? Did you not keep the schedule because of errors in scheduling, fatigue, or unexpected interferences? Did you plan enough restoration and leisure time into your schedule? Looking at the example of the weekly schedule in Chart 6, you can see that not enough restorative time was built into each day and that there is room to delegate tasks, such as picking up kids from practice by arranging a carpool with other families.

Your answers to the questions in Table 1 will help you as you create your schedule for the following week or month. If you noticed that whenever you paired grocery shopping with laundry you were more tired and accomplished fewer other tasks, try putting grocery shopping and laundry on different days, and note any changes in task accomplishment or fatigue level. If you noticed that your symptoms were always worse on Wednesday and that you often scheduled a lot tasks on Tuesdays, try changing your schedule around, and note any change in symptoms on Wednesday. If you are using any disease-modifying medications, you might notice that, on the days

Table 1:

The days of the week or times of the day that I was noticeably more fatigued were _____
The following daily combination of activities were difficult to accomplish together _____ _____
The following daily combination of activities was a successful combination of tasks and activities _____ _____
These patterns occurred between my symptoms and activities _____
I was unable to accomplish the following task because _____
I was unable to keep to my schedule on _____ days because _____
Did I plan enough restoration and leisure time into my schedule? _____

that you get your shot or the day following a weekly shot, you may experience more fatigue. By being aware of these symptoms, you can try and modify the day of the week or time of day that you do this task.

Adapting your schedule

There will be days and weeks when, for reasons out of your control, you will need to adjust your schedule. It is important to remember that these weekly and monthly schedules are only guides; they are not written in stone and can be changed if you feel the need. At the last minute, a meeting or appointment of yours may be cancelled and rescheduled for 2 weeks later, a child can get sick, or your symptoms of

Chart 6
Example of a completed weekly calendar

	SUN	MON	TUES	WED	THURS	FRI	SAT
7AM		Wake up/eat breakfast	Wake up/eat breakfast	Wake up/eat breakfast	Wake up/eat breakfast	Wake up/eat breakfast	Wake up/eat breakfast
8AM		Drop kids off at school/go to work	Drop kids off at school/go to work	Drop kids off at school/go to work	Drop kids off at school/go to work	Drop kids off at school/go to work	Wake up/shower
9AM		Work	Work	Work	Work	Work	Eat breakfast, drive Danielle to ballet
10AM	Wake up/shower	Work	Meeting at work	Work	Staff meeting	Work	
11AM	Eat breakfast	Break to stretch	Break to stretch	Break to stretch	Break to stretch	Break to stretch	
12PM	Go to church	Work	Work	Work	Doctor's appointment	Work	Pick up Danielle; mall with Danielle

Continued on next page

Chart 6, continued

	SUN	MON	TUES	WED	THURS	FRI	SAT
1PM	Work	Work	Work	Doctor's appointment	Work	Shopping	
2PM	Lunch w/ Jean	Work	Work	Work	Doctor's appointment	Work	Shopping
3PM		Work	Work	Work	Go for a walk along the beach	Work	Grocery shopping
4PM		Work	Work	Work	Pick Robert up from school, bring him to hockey	Work	RELAX
5PM		Pick up Danielle from track practice	Drive home	Drive home	Watch Robert's hockey		Make dinner
6PM	Start making dinner	Eat dinner	Eat dinner	Eat dinner	Watch Robert's hockey	Have a snack	Eat dinner

Chart 6, *continued*

	SUN	MON	TUES	WED	THURS	FRI	SAT
7PM			Pilates		Watch Robert's hockey	Pilates	
8PM	Eat dinner			Help Robert w/ his project	Grab quick dinner w/ Robert		
9PM		Shower/ TV	Shower/ TV	Shower/ TV	Shower/ TV	Dinner	Watch a movie
10PM	Go to sleep	Go to sleep	Go to sleep	Go to sleep	Go to sleep	Shower	
11PM						Go to sleep	
12AM							Go to sleep
1AM							
2AM							
Tasks not completed					Watching	Left work	Watching the

Continued on next page

Chart 6, *continued*

	SUN	MON	TUES	WED	THURS	FRI	SAT
Comments	I had a very relaxed day today. I'm feeling good.	Feeling good today.			Was pretty hot out today—not best day for the beach. I the rink I started feeling dizzy and had blurry vision. Had someone else drive Robert home.	Vision still very blurry today. Left work At early.	I was so tired today I fell asleep at 8:30 pm. Did a little too much today.

multiple sclerosis can be particularly bad. By having a monthly schedule, you can look ahead to identify a particularly rough week, and you can adjust your weekly schedule to make it less packed. At other times, you may experience a day when your symptoms worsen unexpectedly. Although it may change what you accomplish in your schedule that day, you have the ability to look ahead and see where you can adjust your future schedule to complete the tasks that you had been unable to accomplish on the day when your symptoms were worse than usual. If you were supposed to have done yard work that day, yet, later in the week, you had scheduled a movie day, you could watch the movie instead, and try fitting yard work into the schedule later in the week.

Looking at the completed monthly calendar (Chart 7), you can see that, in Week 2, your husband will be away, which means that all of the childcare responsibilities will fall on you, and, in Week 3, you have scheduled a lot of appointments. By knowing this in advance, you can perhaps arrange for help in carpooling the kids, plan to order take out, or make meals ahead of time to reheat. During Week 3, you may want to ask your husband or someone else to take the kids to their appointment, and knowing that you will be away for the weekend at a soccer tournament may require putting other tasks at different times during the week. By seeing this visually in advance, there will be no surprise of "How am I going to do all this?"

To adapt your schedule with ease, it may be helpful to create your calendar on a computer so that changes can be easily made or you may want to write activities in pencil so that they can be erased. It may also be helpful to keep your monthly schedule on a dry erase board so that the monthly schedules can be easily changed and adapted and so that

Chart 7
Example of a completed monthly calendar

SUN	MON	TUES	WED	THURS	FRI	SAT
	1 Labor Day	2 Pilates class	3	4	5	6 Family party at the cottage
7	8 Everyone's passports need to be renewed	9 Pilates class	10 Husband on business trip	11 Back to school night; husband on business trip	12 Husband home from business trip	13 Soccer game
14	15	16 Pilates class	17 Danielle and Robert dentist appointment 2:30pm	18 Neurologist appointment	19 Soccer tournament in Maine	20 Soccer tournament in Maine
21 Soccer tournament in Maine	22	23 Pilates class	24	25	26	27 Soccer game
28 Maya's 7th Birthday	29	30 Pilates is cancelled				

all family members, roommates, etc. know what is happening and when. You may even be surprised if you do this, that others may start taking on tasks themselves without you even asking.

A practical schedule is a balanced schedule

Every person is unique, with different life roles and responsibilities. The importance of a particular task will vary from person to person and can change from day to day. If you want to stick to your schedule, you must create a schedule balanced between activities that have to get done and activities that you enjoy doing. Also, to be able to fit everything in, you need to balance your schedule between tasks that are necessary but are tiring to do, with tasks that help you feel rejuvenated when completed. It is important to keep in mind that some tasks that "need to get done" can be delegated to family and friends. Reorganize your schedule to match your priorities with your interests in Chart 2.

My life in a dresser

Before creating your next schedule, think of your list of things to do as a dresser in which you keep your clothes. In the top drawer of your dresser, put all of the items that you *"have to do."* These are important tasks and activities that must get done during the week. Make sure to put them in your schedule first so they have priority. In the second drawer, include the items that you *"need to do."* These items can be put off for a while—but are still important. In the third drawer, include activities that you *"want to do."* In the fourth drawer, include restorative activities, and, last, in the bottom drawer, include the tasks that you can *give to someone else to do.* Then, when planning your daily, weekly, and monthly schedules, think about getting dressed in the morning. To be dressed appropriately, you select clothes from each drawer. Similarly, when selecting items to "dress your schedule," you need to select activities from each drawer to have a balanced and appropriate schedule for yourself.

As you begin the dresser activity, look at the tasks, routines, and activities that you have already identified that you do on a daily, weekly, or monthly basis. Remember to include the activities you do for yourself (self-care activities such as bathing, dressing, medication, grooming, etc); activities you do for others (children, spouses, significant others, siblings, parents, or grandparents, pets, etc.); activities that you do to maintain your home (grocery shopping, laundry, cleaning, yard work, repairs, etc); activities you do for work (transportation to and from, work brought home, business trips, regularly scheduled activities done at work which you know tire you out, etc); and last, but NOT least, activities that are enjoyable (hobbies, reading, movies, creating nice meals, etc.). Use Chart 8 to begin noting the different activities and in which drawer they should go.

Chart 8
My activities and the drawers in which they belong

Activity	Top drawer *Have to do*	Second drawer *Need to do*	Third drawer *Want to do*	Bottom drawer *Give to someone else to do*
Self-care				
Care of others				

Continued on next page

Chart 8, *continued*

Activity	Top drawer *Have to do*	Second drawer *Need to do*	Third drawer *Want to do*	Bottom drawer *Give to someone else to do*
Home maintenance				
Work related				

Chart 8, *continued*

Activity	Top drawer _Have to do_	Second drawer _Need to do_	Third drawer _Want to do_	Bottom drawer _Give to someone else to do_
Leisure				
Restorative activities				

Summary

To manage your fatigue and fit in all of the important things in your life, you need to plan appropriately and be flexible in your plans. The way you schedule your time can affect your daily symptoms and levels of energy.

Proper planning will help you manage your fatigue and help you to adjust to unexpected circumstances, such as variations in your symptoms and changes in your plans. Make sure to create a balanced and manageable schedule for yourself. Include activities that you enjoy and want to do, not only activities that have to get done, and remember to include restorative activities. Don't be afraid to delegate tasks to others, especially those that are most tiring. Lastly, enjoy the process. Decorate your schedule in a way that is visually pleasing to you so that it is something to which you want to refer, and take the time to acknowledge all that you accomplish each day. Nothing in time management is more satisfying than crossing things off the list! In the next chapter, you will look at how your environments can impact your energy levels.

7

Do I Have to Go Upstairs Again? How Your Environments Tire You Out

Megan Boyce, OTS, and
Nancy Lowenstein, OTR

It's not only activities and keeping a busy schedule that can wear you out. The places in which you spend time can also affect how much energy you use during the day. It is important to consider how your different environments are set up and the impact that the setup has on your energy level. The conditions of the environment can make your activities easier or harder to perform. You can change or adapt your existing environments to create spaces that make your activities easier to do and help you to better manage your fatigue.

In this chapter, we will explore simple environment modifications for your home and other places that you spend your time: where you work, shop, worship, and spend time with family and friends.

In this chapter we will discuss
- How environments tire people out
- What about environments can be changed to help manage fatigue
- Where you do important activities and how your environment makes your activities tiring
- How to set up workspaces: ergonomics
- What can be difficult about making changes to environments

How environments tire people out

It is important to take a close look at the spaces in which you live, work, socialize, and interact throughout the day so that you can see how these spaces make your activities more or less fatiguing and how they affect your overall energy level. The setup of these spaces can add to the energy demands of an activity. Consider the following example of environment adding to fatigue: Megan lives in a one-bedroom apartment; Pam lives in a two-story home. Who will use more energy keeping her home clean?

Pam's larger home has more area to clean. Pam will use more energy carrying supplies over longer distances. She will also have to walk and carry supplies up and down the stairs. When cleaning her apartment, Megan will have less area to clean, shorter distances to carry supplies, and no trips up and down the stairs. Megan's energy level will be less depleted than Pam's during this common activity because of the environment in which the activity is performed.

The size of your home is one aspect of the environment that impacts your level of fatigue. Other factors maybe the temperature, noise, or lighting (see Chart 1). One obvious solution to these space problems would be to completely change environments, either by moving to a smaller home or renovating, but these are often not viable options. Other modifications that can help to lessen the burden of fatigue are simpler to implement than an environmental overhaul.

Chart 1 The space I am looking at is the _____

Is it ...

Too hot?	Y	N
Too loud?	Y	N
Too stressful?	Y	N
Too bright?	Y	N
Too far?	Y	N
Too high?	Y	N
Too big?	Y	N

What about environments can be changed to help manage fatigue?

You may not be aware of aspects of your commonly used spaces that may have an impact on your fatigue level. Certainly, size is the one that is most evident; however, other aspects of your space may affect fatigue and will not require a large outlay of money to change, with a good payback in terms of feeling less tired. This sectiion will explore different aspects of your environment and how these factors may impact your fatigue.

Temperature

Is it too hot?

Spending time and doing activities in a room that is too hot can increase fatigue. Keep in mind that heat and increased core body temperature are major contributors to fatigue. It is important to figure out the best temperature for you to live in and to modify your environment to help maintain that temperature. You may live with someone who has different temperature needs than you do; in this case, it is important to find a middle ground for everyone involved. It may require one person to wear a sweater or one to wear short sleeves to feel comfortable, but these compromises are possible.

How to beat the heat

Consider installing an air conditioning unit or fans in your home or car. Even air conditioning one frequently used room can be helpful. You can figure out which room is the one you use the most and arrange to do as many tasks as possible in this space. Hanging window coverings to block excess sunlight from entering and heating your home, office, or vehicle is a very effective way to beat the heat. I remember my mother closing all the curtains on the sunny side of the house in the summer during the daytime and opening them up at night. In this way, the sun's hot rays did not heat up the room. Consider using breathable materials on chairs and furniture. As nice as leather is to see and keep clean, it does not breathe and can trap heat, transferring heat to your body when you sit on it. This is especially true in a car, where leather seats can become especially hot. Trade these materials for cotton or other breathable cloth materials. You don't have to buy new furniture or a new car; instead, you can have slipcovers made, get a large sheet and put it on the furniture, buy a breathable cover for your car seat, or even use a towel to sit on.

Other ways to beat the heat

If it is not possible to control the temperature of your environment, think about other strategies. For example, you may want to schedule activities during cooler times of the day. If your home is hottest in the afternoon, consider cooking dinner in the morning when the kitchen is coolest and then reheating the meal later before serving. Outdoor activity may also be scheduled depending on when it is coolest; doing errands in the morning or evening hours when the temperature is lower may be best. If you can't reschedule a task to a cooler time, consider wearing a cooling vest or a cool cloth on the back of your neck to keep your body temperature down. Wear light-colored and loose clothing made of breathable materials, usually natural fibers or blends.

In the box on the next page, write down the spaces that you frequently use that are too hot and brainstorm about some possible solutions to beating the heat.

NOISE

Is it too loud?

The noise level in your environment can affect your energy level. Loud and irritating noises, like the sound of the lawn

Spaces that may be too hot	Solutions to beating the heat

mower or honking car horns, may stress your nervous system and contribute to fatigue. You may not be aware that sounds are bothering you, like the hum of electronics equipment, until you remove them from your environment.

How to lower the volume

Decreasing the stress and fatigue caused by too much noise in your environment may be as simple as turning off or lowering the volume on the television or other electronics. If you cannot get rid of noises, consider installing a music player, nature-sounds machine, water statue, or white-noise machine in your home or office to help replace stressful noises with calming sounds. You can copy the effect of a white-noise machine by using other consistent noises, such as the sound of a fan or air conditioner. Use calming sounds or soft music at home, at work, or in your vehicle to decrease fatigue after completing various activities in these environments. Adding insulation such as carpet and wall fabrics may help decrease the noise entering your environment from street noise, from apartment mates, or between rooms in your home.

Other ways to lower the volume

You may not be able to control the noises in your environment around the clock because of other people and events in the environment. Consider working out a schedule with housemates, designating certain hours for noisy activities, like using the hair dryer or television, and other hours for more quiet activities to help you plan ahead for managing your stress. You may want to change environments by going to the library or another quiet location if noises in your environment, such as construction, cannot be controlled and are causing fatigue. Having kids in the house is noise producing in itself. They may have noisy games and toys or shout and yell a lot. Make a "noisy" and "quiet" play time, put the noisy toys away after dinner; make a no-shouting rule and create a noise zone, perhaps even outside. You may find that everyone benefits from this "quieter" time.

Spaces that may be too noisy	Solutions to decreasing the noise

Stress

Is your space causing stress?

Environments themselves may cause stress and frustration that can increase your fatigue. Disorganization, clutter, broken tools, and cramped spaces may heighten your stress level. Stress uses up emotional and physical energy, increasing feelings of fatigue.

How to stop environmental stress

If small and cramped spaces are causing stress, consider reorganizing your space, getting rid of things that you no longer need or use, and purchasing storage containers to help control the clutter in your home, car, or work environments. A good rule of thumb is that if you haven't used it, looked at it, or worn it in a year, you can safely get rid of it. If you are saving toys, knickknacks, or broken equipment, fix them, give them away, or throw them out. Create good habits for clearing out the junk. When the mail comes, immediately sort it, and throw out the junk mail; have a space to put the bills and catalogues and decide immediately what to do with each piece of mail. If you have a desk that is piled high with papers, start with one pile, corner, or a desk drawer, and clean that first; then move on to the next pile and so on until you have finished that section. This may take several weeks to accomplish, so keep your eye on the prize at the end—a stress-free space. Develop color-coding filing systems, so your bills are one color, medical information is another color, etc., and make a place for everything. This won't happen in a week, but it's worth the time in the long run. Great books have been written about how to declutter your spaces, but check the book out of the library so you don't have something else to clutter your bookshelves when you finish reading it!

Other ways to stop the stress

Your kitchen may be organized but may still be too small to cook in with someone else. Or you may find it difficult to get ready in the morning if you are sharing bathroom space with other family members. Scheduling activities that have to be done in limited spaces can help to get rid of the stress caused by cramped or cluttered environments. In the box below, write down the spaces that you frequently use that are stressful or cluttered and ways to make these spaces better.

Spaces that may be too stressful or cluttered	Solutions to taming the stress or clutter

Lighting

Is it too bright? Is there poor light?

The lighting where you spend time and do activities can make your activities more or less fatiguing. Bright lights, glare, or older types of fluorescent lights can overstimulate your nervous system, causing headaches and eye strain, and can contribute to an increase in fatigue. Having too little light or indirect light makes it hard for you to see during tasks, such as reading; having the wrong lighting can also cause stress and fatigue.

How to right the light

Make sure that there is enough light for you to see easily while doing activities. Consider using task lighting, such as a desk lamp for writing or a book light for reading, to avoid eyestrain. You can also adjust the brightness of a computer screen or use a glare shield to decrease eye fatigue. Sunshades in your home, car, or office can also lessen excessive light and glare. Flickering fluorescent bulbs can be upgraded to those using electronic ballasts to eliminate the flicker. You may find natural light, soft light bulbs, or candles more relaxing than other lighting, and you can use these in your environment to control your fatigue.

Where you place objects is also important. If you place a computer monitor or TV screen in front of a window, you will have to fight off the bright glare of the light that is behind the object. So, use a shade, curtain, or blinds on the window or move the TV or computer screen so that the window is behind or to the side of it.

Other ways to right the light

You may not have direct control over the lighting used at work or in public facilities. Consider talking with the individuals in charge of these environments to discuss the benefits that all individuals can gain from ergonomic lighting: fewer headaches, less eyestrain, more energy, and greater

Spaces that have lighting issues	Solutions to resolving the lighting problems

productivity. In the box on the previous page, write down the spaces that you frequently use that have lighting issues and ways to solve these problems.

HEIGHT

Is it too far or too high?
Doing activities in your home, at work, or in other environments often involves tasks such as walking, reaching, or bending, which can use up a lot of energy. The way your environment is organized can require including more or fewer of these tiring tasks. You may have to reach for items in closets or cabinets or carry supplies throughout your home, but the way you organize your space can help you to save energy on these tasks.

How to fight the far and high
To save your energy that would be used up by bending, reaching, and carrying supplies, organize your home so that the items you use most often are the easiest to access. Consider organizing all storage areas, such as closets, dressers, pantries, garages, and your home office, so that popular items are easy to access and items are stored close to where they will be used. In the kitchen, have the dishes and pans that are used most frequently on the shelves that are most accessible—that is, between your waist and shoulder height—therefore, limiting how much you have to bend and reach. Put items on open shelves versus closed cabinets (Image 1). In addition to organizing items according to their frequency of use, try to store items within each room close to the area or surface where you will use them, such as storing pans in cabinets close to the stove. You may consider not storing frequently used items in cabinets, but, instead,

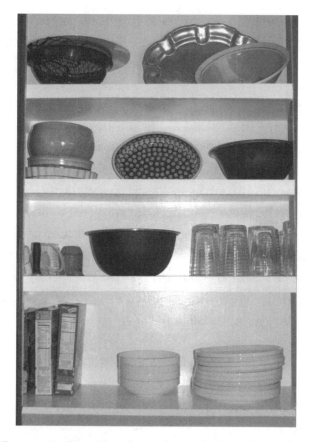

*Image 1. Open cupboards make reaching for
dishes and other items easy.*

keeping your most-used pots and pans on the stove itself
(Image 2). A low-hanging pot rack can also be used, as long
as it isn't so high and far away as to require a huge reach.

In the shower, store items on wall shelves instead of
along the lip of the shower or tub. Another energy-saving
strategy for storage areas is to limit stacking items on top
of each other, which requires you to move several items to
access those on the bottom of the stack. If necessary, stack
items with those needed most often on the top, or use a
vertical storage system or pullout drawers. To save energy

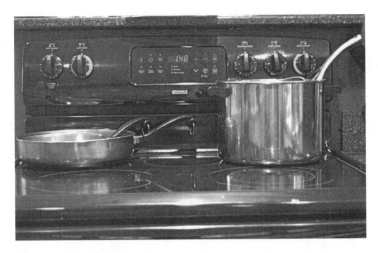

Image 2. Sometimes it's simpler to leave the pans that you use most often right on the stovetop.

while doing laundry, you may want to use separate laundry baskets for darks and lights, ask family members to take their laundry to the washer, and keep all laundry supplies at an easy level for access.

To decrease walking and carrying of items from room to room, store items throughout the home in the area in which they will be used. For example, instead of carrying cleaning supplies throughout your home, store a bottle of bathroom cleaner and paper towels under each bathroom sink. For cleaning a multistory home, you may want to have a set of supplies on each floor to eliminate the need to carry objects up and down the stairs.

Other ways to fight the far and high
In addition to organizing your home as already described, you can save energy by creating workstations at an easily accessible height, again limiting bending and reaching. If you have a front-loading washer, consider using cinder blocks to raise the machine and decrease the need to bend

when loading the laundry. For working in the kitchen with high counters, you may want to sit on a high stool so that your elbows can be relaxed and bent along your sides. In the box below, write down the spaces that you frequently use that need reorganizing as far as distance and height, and develop some solutions to these problems.

Spaces that may be too far or high	Solutions to these problems

SIZE

Is it too big?

Large spaces or moving large objects may also contribute to your energy loss. You may have to move furniture around your home or office to access items in cabinets or to open doors. You may also have to rearrange while cleaning. This extra work makes an already busy day more difficult and uses up your energy. Your space may be so large that you need to move around a lot to access supplies or complete a task.

How to battle the big

For items in your environments that have to be moved frequently, consider making them easier to move by putting them on wheels or removing friction surfaces, such as thick rugs, from underneath them. You can put furniture on casters or on gliders to move them easily; these can be found in most hardware stores. If your house is large, try to use only a few rooms that are close together. Think about your day and what you will need when you come downstairs in the morning so that you don't have to make extra trips back up the stairs. Keep duplicate items in different rooms so that you don't have to go looking for them. Also, look at rearranging a large space into smaller work or sitting areas within the room. This will make the room seem cozier while at the same time decrease the amount of moving around that you need to do.

Other ways to battle the big

Big spaces such as malls, grocery stores, and big-box stores can seem overwhelming, and the thought of going there may be tiring. Most of these places now offer electric scooters with baskets on them. You may have to ask at the service desk for a key, but it is well worth it in terms of energy saved for more fun things. You needn't be embarrassed to use these devices, and the myth that, if you aren't walking then you are giving into your disease, is just that, a myth. In the box below, write down any spaces that are

Spaces that may be too large or include objects	Solutions to dealing with BIG

large or large objects that you need to move and solutions to these issues.

The places you spend your time

Think about the environments you live in: home, work, school, public facilities, recreational parks, and places you shop or go to with friends. Use Chart 2 to make a list of your unique environments and their shortfalls. To help you brainstorm, consider what you do on a typical weekday and weekend and where these activities take place: consider errands, social activities, work, transportation, etc.

Chart 2

Evaluating problems in my environment

My environments   **The problems**

Where you do important activities and how your environment makes your activities tiring

By now, you have a better understanding of how your space can have an impact on you in many ways. So far, you have listed your environments and where they fall short. Now, it is time to think about ways to make them work better for you and others in your life. You will find that the changes you make will have a positive impact not only on you, but also on others who share these spaces.

1. Look at the list of your environments you made earlier in this chapter.
2. For each environment, list the activities that you do in the environment that are fatiguing. For example, in the kitchen, you may list washing dishes, putting away dishes, cooking, cleaning, and putting away groceries.
3. Ask yourself why the activity in this environment is fatiguing. Use Chart 1 on page 103 "Is it . . ." to help you figure out how the environment tires you out.
4. Then, list ways to change your environment to make it less fatiguing. Look in the section listing ways to change environments for solutions that will work for you in your environments. You may want to do this activity with the other people who share the space, as they may have some good ideas as well.

Take a look at Chart 3 for an example of how to complete this analysis of your environment. Chart 4 provides you with an environment—your kitchen at home—and starts you off with some activities that you might perform in your kitchen. Now you fill in the rest.

Chart 3
A completed chart of activities and environment

Environment: kitchen at home

Activities in the environment: washing dishes, putting dishes away, cooking, cleaning and putting away groceries

Factors contributing to fatigue	Contributors to fatigue in your environment	Ways to change the environment
Is it too hot?	Yes. When I use the dishwasher, oven, or stove, my kitchen gets uncomfortably hot.	Use a fan, open windows, or install an a/c unit to help keep the kitchen temperature more comfortable for cooking.
Is it too loud?	Yes. When people turn on the TV in the living room, the sound travels into the kitchen.	Develop a schedule for the house so that cooking and watching TV don't happen at the same time.
Is it too stressful?	Yes. It is hard to cook when other people are trying to use the kitchen..	Develop a schedule for when people will use the kitchen
Is it too bright?	Yes. The overhead lights in my kitchen hurt my eyes.	Turn lights off in the kitchen and instead use natural light coming through windows, lights on in another room, or under the counter lights.

Chart 3, *continued*
A completed chart of activities and environment

Environment: kitchen at home

Activities in the environment: washing dishes, putting dishes away, cooking, cleaning and putting away groceries

Factors contributing to fatigue	Contributors to fatigue in your environment	Ways to change the environment
Is it too far?	Yes. My pantry is not in my kitchen, and I have to walk back and forth down the hallway to get supplies.	Set up the kitchen to make supplies more accessible, storing items used every day, like cereal, on the counter and the pots used most often on the stovetop.
Is it too high?	Yes. The counter is too high for me to sit while I'm working in the kitchen.	Organize workstations with help, gathering all of the supplies in a designated work area before starting to cook. Use a stool in the kitchen to sit while preparing meals.
Is it too big?	Yes. I have to move the kitchen trashcan to open the broom closet.	Put the trashcan on a piece of wood with wheels so it is easier to move.

Chart 4
A blank chart for evaluating a workspace from an ergonomic perspective

Environment: kitchen at home

Activities in the environment: washing dishes, putting dishes away, cooking, cleaning and putting away groceries

Factors contributing to fatigue	Contributors to fatigue in your environment	Ways to change the environment
Is it too far?		
Is it too high?		
Is it too big?		

Chart 4, continued
A blank chart for evaluating a workspace from an ergonomic perspective

Environment: kitchen at home

Activities in the environment: washing dishes, putting dishes away, cooking, cleaning and putting away groceries

Factors contributing to fatigue	Contributors to fatigue in your environment	Ways to change the environment
Is it too far?		
Is it too high?		
Is it too big?		

Setting up spaces: ergonomics

Ergonomics is the practice of setting up your space to complete activities in the most efficient manner, reducing stress and strain on your body, and, thus, making your activities less fatiguing. Using ergonomic principles helps you to think about how your body does specific tasks and still maintains a comfortable and relaxed position. By setting up spaces ergonomically, you can avoid repetitive stress injuries such as carpal tunnel syndrome, learn to support your body properly, and, in the end, use less energy during the task.

Chart 5

Identify the spaces you use that need an ergonomic overhaul

Spaces in which I sit for a long time

_____

_____

_____

Spaces in which I stand for a long time

_____

_____

_____

Spaces in which I regularly do a task

_____

_____

_____

Where to use ergonomics

Consider making changes to the many workspaces within your environments. Workspaces are anywhere you sit or stand for an extended period of time while working on a task. These workspaces include a desk at work or in your home office, the kitchen while cooking, the laundry room while folding laundry, or even your car when driving.

What are the principles of ergonomics?

The main ergonomic principles are to keep your body comfortable and relaxed. Standards have been developed that enable people to use the most ergonomically correct methods to perform a task. Below you will find the main ergonomic principles for when you are sitting and standing.

Sitting

- Make sure that your feet are flat on floor. If they don't reach, then place your feet on a foot stool.
- Keep your knees at a 90° to 110° angle relative to the back of your thighs.
- Keep your hips at about a right angle, slightly open.
- Support your lower back, using a small pillow or rolled towel to provide lumbar support if your chair lacks a built-in support.
- Keep your shoulders relaxed. It is amazing how often you hunch up and tighten your shoulders and don't even know it. Tight muscles take more energy than relaxed muscles do to maintain in that position.
- Keep your elbows relaxed and close to your body. This is the natural position of the arm.

continued on next page

Sitting, *continued*

- Keep your forearms supported on the table or desk or armrests and parallel to the floor. When your forearms are supported, the muscles aren't working as hard and you can write or type for a longer period of time.
- Keep your head and neck aligned with your spine, not jutted forward or looking down. You may have to adjust your computer monitor to help with this (Images 3 and 4).
- Keep your wrists in a neutral position. That is not bent up or down.
- Take a small break every hour.

Standing

- Find a counter or table that is a good height.
- Do not hunch over or bend at the waist.
- Put equal weight on both feet or, to relieve lower back pain, stand with one foot slightly raised on a step.
- Keep your shoulders relaxed.
- Keep your elbows close to your body.
- Keep your forearms supported and about parallel to the floor. This may be more difficult in a standing position, so, if you can't keep your forearms supported, relax them to your sides every 15 minutes or so.
- Keep your head and neck aligned with your spine, not jutted forward or looking down.
- Keep your wrists in a neutral position. That is not

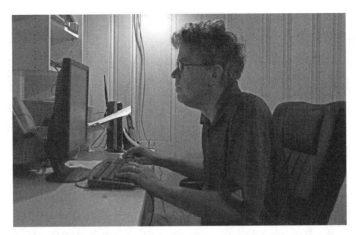

Image 3. Note the position of the hands and forearms as they reach for the keyboard. The head is looking down at the screen, and the shoulders are hunched because the armrests are too high. Holding this position for more than 10 minutes will cause the muscles to begin to tire.

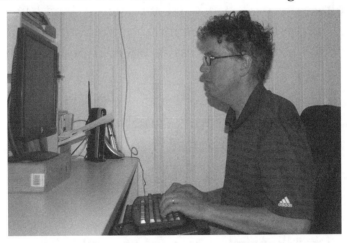

Image 4. Note the better position of the arms with the keyboard and the armrests lowered. With the monitor raised, the head is in a better position, allowing the person to sit up higher and not hunch over. In this position, the muscles are more supported, and the person can sit for longer. Don't forget that, even if you're sitting in the proper position, you will still need to take stretch breaks.

Driving

How many times have you been driving and realized that you were gripping the wheel, your neck and shoulders were tense, and your back hurt? (Image 5) When you drive, do you take advantage of the lumbar support in your car seat? Do you set the seat or the headrest to the right height? Do you hold the steering wheel correctly? If you are not positioned properly, driving a car can steal energy. So, the next time you are in your car, before you start driving, check your seat height and distance from the pedals; the back of your head should rest on the back support. If your car seat doesn't have a built-in lumbar support, you can fold a small towel and place it behind the small of your back. Lastly, support your elbows on the armrests, and place your hands on the steering wheel at 3 and 9 o'clock, keeping your elbows relaxed and slightly bent (Image 6). Once you have found a comfortable position, you will find that driving is not so stressful on your body and not as exhausting.

What can be difficult about making changes to your environments?

So far, in this chapter, you have learned ways to change your spaces to make activities you do use up less energy. But, initially making these changes may itself use up a lot of energy! Remember to pace yourself when making changes to your environments. Even making one change, such as adding a fan to a heated environment, can make an important difference in helping you save energy. Don't feel as if you have to make many changes to achieve a benefit or that all of the changes to your environments need to be made immediately. Additionally, changes don't need to

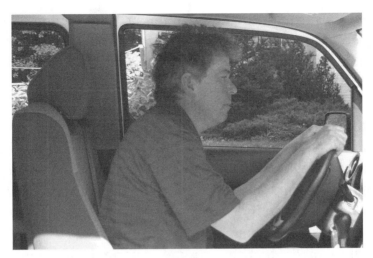

Image 5. Poor positioning in the car.
The body is not adequately supported.

be costly; you may need to be creative. You may also consider asking a friend or relative to help you make changes
or hiring help to complete more large-scale and fatiguing

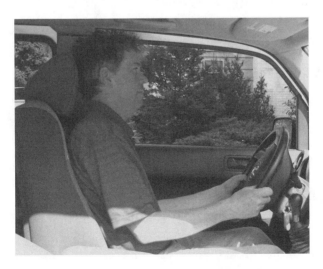

Image 6. Proper position is achieved by using
the seat back, head rest, and arm rest to support
the body while driving.

changes, such as moving furniture or reorganizing entire closets. Money may also be a concern when making changes to your environment. Many quick fixes use materials that you may already have around your home, such as using books under your feet instead of purchasing a foot rest. The appearance of your home, office, or other environments may also be a consideration. You will need to find a balance between making your environment easier to live in and maintaining a space that you enjoy and that is functional. For environments in which you may not be in control of making changes, you may need to advocate or convince others that changes are important and would be beneficial to many people. You may need to engage coworkers or contact local support groups or agencies to connect with other people in your area who are advocating for common changes. An occupational therapist can be a good professional to evaluate your space for ergonomics, safety, and energy conservation.

How to make changes more easily

- Pace yourself
- Consider asking for help
- Use materials that are already in your environment to save money
- Balance functionality of your space and appearance
- Advocate to make changes in public areas
- Talk with other people in similar situations for ideas and support

---

Summary

When working to manage your fatigue, keep in mind that the environments in which you spend your time can make activities more or less fatiguing. Simple changes to your environments can help you to save energy and feel better. Consider the aspects of your environments at home, work, school, and places you shop or spend time with family and friends. Think about the light, temperature, noise, stress, the size of the area, and the size of objects in the environment. Think about the activities you do in these environments and how aspects of the environments make your activities more fatiguing. Brainstorm solutions to help manage your environments and your fatigue. Also remember that setting up ergonomic workstations can help you to feel better and less fatigued. Pace yourself when making changes to your environments. You may need to advocate for changes in public spaces or recruit help for large-scale changes. In the next chapter, you will examine ways to simplify specific activities.

8

Ways to Simplify
Activities and Tasks

Nancy Lowenstein, OTR

A friend of mine tells a story about baking a ham. Whenever she bakes a ham, she cuts off both ends. She has been doing this her whole life because she thought it was necessary to cook the ham correctly. One year, she asked her mother, who had taught her this technique, why she did this. The answer: the ham didn't fit into her baking pan and that was the only way to make it fit! I start with this story to make the point that we often do things a certain way without thinking about why or whether it is the most efficient way to accomplish the task.

Our lives are filled with lots of tasks and activities that we have been doing a certain way without thinking about why we do it that way. Sometimes we do a job in a certain way because that is how we were taught to do it (like my friend and her ham); sometimes it is the only way you can think of to do the activity (because you have always done it that way). However, the way you are doing some common activities may not be the most efficient way and, therefore, may be contributing to your fatigue.

In this chapter, you will look at different common activities and specific ways to change them, as well as look at some simple gadgets and tools that you can purchase to help make activities easier.

In this chapter you will learn
- Ways to simplify common activities
- Ways to change habits
- How to delegate tasks

Ways to simplify

In Chapter 3, you learned principles of looking at yourself, the activity, or the environment to change the way you are doing an activity. Look at the listing of common activities in this chapter, and use the suggestions as starting points to think about changes that fit your particular needs (Table 1).

Changing habits

Habits are useful in that they allow us to be able to complete tasks without thinking about them. Imagine having to stop and think about where the ignition is every time you get into your car, or how to hold your toothbrush. By creat-

Table 1: Common activities and ways in which you can change them

Activity	Change yourself	Change activity	Change environment
Showering	Strengthen quadriceps Improve balance	Shower when you have more energy or at night.	Use grab bars, a tub seat and handheld shower.
		Use a terrycloth robe instead of towel to dry your body. Sit on toilet to dry off. Change to different shampoo or soap containers that are easier to open, close, and hold	Remodel bathroom with walk-in shower stall with built-in bench.
Dressing	Stretch your arms and legs to be able to reach behind your back, bring legs up, etc.	Gather all of your clothes together before dressing. Wear clothing without small fasteners. Use elastic shoelaces for shoes or shoes with Velcro or that slip on. Use adaptive equipment so that you don't have to bend.	Put a firm chair in your room to sit on when dressing instead of standing or sitting on the edge of the bed. Make sure clothing is within easy reach in drawers or closets.

Continued on next page

Table 1: Common activities and ways in which you can change them, *continued*

Activity	Change yourself	Change activity	Change environment
Grooming	Strengthen your arms, wrists and hands. Work on balance.	Build up handles on toothbrush, comb, brush, and razor for easier grip. Use smaller containers of toothpaste, shave cream, etc.	Sit down in front of a mirror instead of standing.
Toileting	Strengthen your legs, work on sitting balance.	Pull clothing up over your knee before standing. Make sure toilet paper is within easy reach.	Put rails around toilet. Use raised toilet seat.
Meal preparation	Work on endurance, leg and arm strength.	Make meal in smaller chunks. Make part of the meal in the morning. Use built-up or large-handled utensils. Gather all ingredients at once. Use prepackaged foods. Use a Crockpot, George Forman grill™. Cook a large portion and freeze	Sit to do the tasks of cutting, putting together ingredients. Ask someone to handle the oven. Create work-stations. Arrange the kitchen so you don't have to bend and reach a lot. Keep items on the counter if you use them frequently.

Table 1: Common activities and ways in which you can change them, *continued*

Activity	Change yourself	Change activity	Change environment
Making the bed	Work on endurance, walking, and balance.	Use lightweight comforters. Make one side of the bed, then move to the other side. Eliminate extra pillows. Teach children to make their beds. Don't make the bed.	Buy sheets for the next larger size of bed. Don't put the bed against the wall. Remove clutter from the floor and surfaces.
Cleaning	Work on endurance, balance, arm strength.	Don't try to clean the whole house or apartment in one day. Clean one or two rooms a week or day and rotate through all the rooms. Hire someone to clean. Give kids chores to do. Use easy cleaners such as Swiffer®.	Have cleaning supplies in each room in which they will be used. Use a robotic vacuum or one that is easy to push (an upright is easier than a canister).

Continued on next page

Table 1: Common activities and ways in which you can change them, *continued*

Activity	Change yourself	Change activity	Change environment
Grocery shopping	Work on endurance, balance, walking.	Make a list, plan meals ahead of time. Ask for light bags and for all items that need refrigeration to be put in bags together so that you can wait until others are there to take the bags out of the car.	Go to the same grocery store. Don't go to a superstore. Use an on-line grocery service, if available. Use the scooter provided by the store.
Mealtime	Work on sitting balance, arm strength, and endurance	Use silverware with large grips or build up your grip with insulation foam for pipes. Use cups with a lid or handle if you have a tremor. Use finger foods. Have others set the table	Use lightweight dishes (not paper). Use contrast under dishes and do not use clear glasses if you have vision problems. Make sure your table is at a good height with a firm chair with armrests.

Table 1: Common activities and ways in which you can change them, *continued*

Activity	Change yourself	Change activity	Change environment
Childcare	Work on balance and upper-extremity strength.	Create a changing space so you can sit down while changing, but still keep your infant or toddler safe. Have toys ready to give infant or toddler when changing them to distract them.	Modify crib so that one side opens out instead of going up and down for easier access. Use Tripp Trapp® chair instead of high chair. Use a lightweight folding stroller.
Laundry	Work on balance, arm strength, and leg strength.	Do more frequent but smaller loads. Don't sort; wash in cold water. Place detergent and fabric softener within easy reach. Use a reacher to take laundry out of a top-loading washer.	Buy front-loading washer and dryer. Use a laundry bag and throw it down the stairs instead of using a basket. Ask family members to take their dirty laundry to the washer. Have a table and chair near the washer and dryer for folding.

ing habits from the tasks we perform every day, we are able to perform them faster and even do other tasks at the same time. For instance, when you dress, you can talk on the phone. Habits help us get through our days much faster. However, the way we do something may not always be the fastest, easiest, or safest way, especially if you have mobility or physical problems due to your multiple sclerosis.

Habits can also be difficult to change because, when you are learning to do a task in a new way, it will take longer until the new way becomes a habit. Humans tend to like familiarity, and change is difficult. However, the payback to changing the way you do something can be doing it safer, easier, or faster.

You may have only one habit that you need to change or you may have many, and it can seem daunting to try and figure out new ways to do something. The familiar is comfortable but, again, may be causing you to expend a lot of energy. On the flip side, you can't change all of your habits at once! So, the best way is to choose one activity that you wish to change and start with that; when that becomes a habit, you can try another and keep on going.

Change who does this activity

Lastly, we hang onto activities for many reasons. One is that you don't think anyone can do it as well as you do it or in the same way that you do it; because doing it yourself makes you feel like a good caregiver; or because it feels that, if you give up too many activities, you are "giving in" to your multiple sclerosis. All of these reasons are valid, but if fatigue is a problem for you, then you are not doing yourself or those around you any good by trying to hang onto everything. As you try to hang onto all of your activities, you do them less well and you feel less positive about yourself because you aren't doing things up to "your standards." However, those around you want to help but may not know how, may be afraid to ask, or may not know what you need. So, now is your time to look at what activities you can give to someone else to do. There is one bit of caution that goes with this; if you give up a task and ask someone else to do it, you have to allow them to do it THEIR way, not yours. If you sort the laundry into colors and whites, but your spouse doesn't, then get cold water detergent, keep out anything that is valuable to you from the wash, and tell your spouse to wash everything in cold water. The laundry will be clean, folded, and put away, and you will not have done it! What a great way to fight fatigue!

Table 2 provides some examples for you to look at regarding who else could do an activity for you. Remember, recruiting children to help is fair game. It teaches them responsibility. It does not mean that you are abdicating your parenting role but, instead, that you are teaching them great life skills. Now it's your turn. Use Table 3 to fill in your own tasks.

Energy-saving assistive devices

Finally, you can find many devices in stores that you go to every day that can help you save your energy. These devices make it easier to do common everyday tasks by assisting with the task, such as a food chopper; by giving more mechanical advantage to the task, such as a can or bottle opener; or by making clean-up easier, such as nonstick pots, pans, and griddles. When you are shopping in the grocery store, department stores, or specialty stores, keep your eyes open for items that may be able to make a

Table 2 Completed chart to examine tasks and who can do them

Task	Currently done by	Could be done by	What do I have to give up to have someone else do this task?	Can I give this up?
Grocery shopping	Me	Husband, sister, mother	They won't use coupons or buy sale items.	Maybe; I will try to let go
Put clean laundry away	Me clean cloths	The children could put away their own put in right places	Clothes may not be	Yes!

Table 3 Blank chart to examine tasks and who completes them

Task	Currently done by	Could be done by	What do I have to give up to have someone else do this task?	Can I give this up?

task easier to accomplish. Especially visit the gadget section of these stores. If you would like to make a task easier and wonder if there is an energy-saving device for this activity, check the Internet or the big-box stores and specialty stores. Many mainstream products are now on the market with ergonomic grips, stay-put bases, and other adaptations to make using them easier than the traditional device. Pictured here (as images 1-8) are some of these devices. I am sure you can find more; you may even have some in your house already that you aren't using, so check those drawers and cabinets!

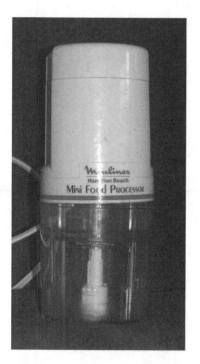

Image 1.
Mini food processor for chopping small amounts of herbs, onion, garlic, and more—a larger one can chop larger amounts and should be kept on the counter.

Image 2. This one-touch can opener requires no hands to use. Just put on the can, touch the button, and watch it go!

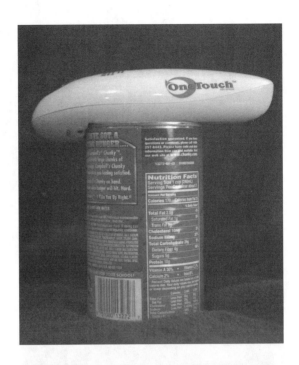

Image 3. A George Forman Grill™ is a quick and easy way to make grilled sandwiches, hamburgers, and other foods and doesn't require flipping the food to cook the other side.

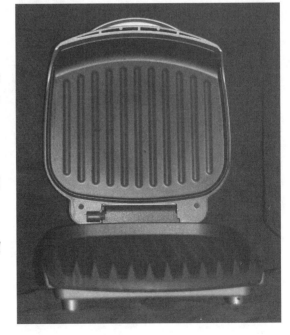

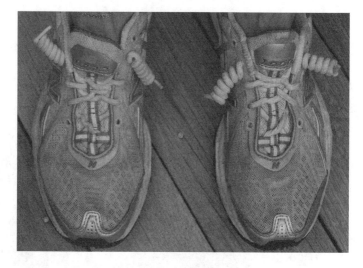

Image 4.
These elastic shoelaces turn sneakers into slip-ons.

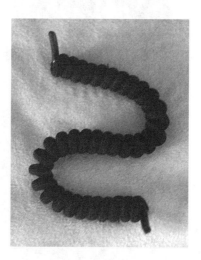

Image 5.
This is a coil of elastic shoelaces before
they are put in the sneaker.

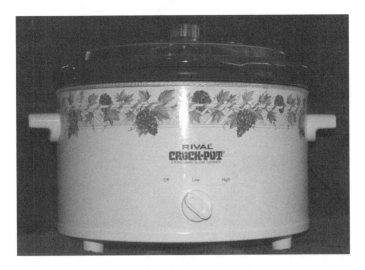

Image 6.
A Crockpot is another easy and efficient way to make delicious meals without expending a lot of energy.

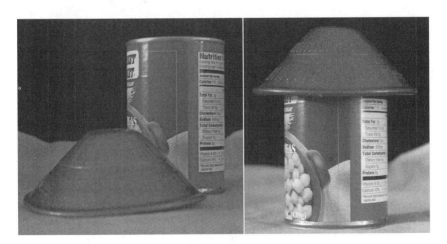

Image 7.
A simple jar gripper can make opening jars easier, even for those with weak hands.

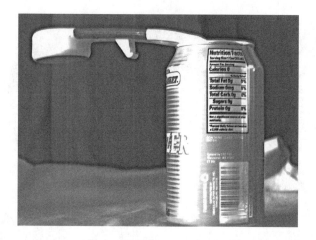

Image 8.
A simple device like this pop-top can opener gives
you more leverage and makes opening cans easier—
and saves a few fingernails as well!

Summary

In this chapter, you looked at very specific activities to get ideas about how to make changes in these activities. Additionally, you looked at the importance of changing existing habits and asking others to help without feeling like you are giving in to your multiple sclerosis. You saw photos of a few of the hundreds of energy-saving assistive devices that are available in the marketplace. Keep your eyes open for them in stores where you shop. Also, ask your physician to refer you for an evaluation by an occupational therapist, who can help you identify different ways to do an activity and equipment that may assist you during a task.

9

How to Make Changes Stick

Daria Rabkin, OTS

Before you make changes, be sure to understand your current habits and why they are not helping you in managing your fatigue. This will help you move forward toward a new life, instead of staying stuck in your current way of doing things. When you do decide to make changes in your life, you must stay on track and continue to follow through until these changes are complete. It is important to develop a mindset that focuses on the changes you wish to make. If you find a reason to change (i.e., decreasing your fatigue), the changes you make will be much more likely to stick. If you actively plan to change (i.e., making small goals for yourself), your goals will be easier to meet. In short, you are more likely to be successful if you have developed a mindset that says you are ready to change.

In this chapter you will learn how to
- Understand your current habits and why they *don't* work
- Develop a "ready-to-change" mindset
- Find a reason to change
- Actively plan to change

Understanding your motivation to change

To alter your lifestyle to implement the suggestions discussed in this book, it is necessary for you to first understand why you want to change. Fatigue is a symptom that may be alleviated by implementing specific strategies into your lifestyle. Although change may seem daunting, it will be beneficial to switch the way you go about your daily routine so that you lessen the effect fatigue has on your well-being. By understanding the effect these changes can have in your daily life, you can become motivated to con-

---

Understanding Your Motivation to Change
- Ask yourself why you want to change
- Understand the results of change
- Become excited about the changes you are making
- Understand the benefits of energy conservation
- Think about the purpose your changes will serve in your life
- Imagine how much better your life will be once the changes are made

---

tinue making your changes and possibly implement other changes to counteract the effects of fatigue. Maintaining a positive attitude by continually realizing the benefits of using these techniques will motivate you to continue to use various techniques throughout your routine.

Your turn

I want to change the way I do things because

By changing behaviors I hope to be able to

I will be excited about making changes by

Be confident

Change can take time—especially when you have already established routines in your daily life. Do not even try to change everything at once, but, instead, choose an area that seems like an easy place to start so that you can experience success. Do not worry if you are not able to implement change immediately or all at once. It is difficult to break routines that have been established for a long time. However, by taking time to analyze your daily and weekly schedules, you can see where to start. Begin with small changes because this will increase your confidence and make you feel more accomplished. Once you begin incorporating ideas, you can add more of them. Some strategies incorporate asking others for help, whereas other strategies rely on you to change the way you do things.

Be Confident
- Have confidence in your ability to change
- Maintain a positive attitude about change
- Understand that change takes time
- Having people who support you increases confidence

Support from other people helps. Letting people know how and why you are trying to make changes in your life will help them understand why you are working so hard; they will support you, as well as help you acknowledge the little accomplishments you make along the way—all of which will boost your confidence.

Your turn

I have confidence in my ability to make changes because

_____

I will be able to stay positive by doing

_____

I will ask for support from

_____

Make your change your mission

Writing a mission statement is a powerful way to help you make a change because it can help you focus on your goals. Keeping focused is important because you do not want to take your eye off your target; if you do, the change will be harder to make. To develop your mission statement, write down what you hope to accomplish, why you want to accomplish it, and how you hope to accomplish it. If you include a target date for the change, your goal will seem more realistic, and you will be more likely to achieve it.

Make Change Your Mission
- Write a mission statement for your change
- Write down what you wish to accomplish, why you want to make the change, how you wish to make the change, and the date by which you want to make the change
- Make your mission into a simple slogan that will remind you of your goal

Once you have written your mission statement, make it into a slogan that you can and will remember, and repeat it to remind yourself of the goal or goals you wish to accomplish. Your slogan can be a fact, an idea, a statement of purpose, or even a question, as long as it is a simple phrase that expresses your reason to change. Keep refining your slogan until you get it down to a simple clear phrase because the objective is for you to have something easy to remember that will remind you of what you are trying to accomplish. Chart 1 shows an example to help you create your mission statement and slogans for every change you may want to make. Put your slogan someplace where you and others can see it everyday. Share your mission and slogan with others, and ask for help in reaching it. Now it's your turn! Use Chart 2 to outline your own goals and how you plan to accomplish them.

Chart 1
Example of a completed goal-setting worksheet

What you want to accomplish	Why you want make a change	How you hope to make the change	Target date for making the change	Your mission statement or slogan
Example: eat less junk food and more "real" food	I want to savor the food; I don't want to fill up on processed foods anymore	Buy healthy food: eat more fruits, vegetables, and nuts; eat in moderation; savor my food	June 30, 2009	Healthy food equals better mood

Chart 2
A blank goal-setting worksheet

What you want to accomplish	Why you want make a change	How you hope to make the change	Target date for making the change	Your mission statement or slogan

Start small

When making changes, it is essential to initially start small. It is too much to drastically change your routine. Begin by implementing one strategy, and, once you have established that strategy in your life, you can begin to implement other changes. Once you are confident in your new ability, you can try to make another change. While evaluating your daily routine and determining the ways you can incorporate energy conservation tips, you can decide what changes will work best for you. By implementing small changes and gradually incorporating more tips into your daily routine, you will gain confidence in your ability to implement and maintain change.

Start Small

- Start by adding small goals, and take it one step at a time
- Continue to add changes as you are able
- Focus on one goal at a time

I will start by choosing the small task of

_____

Set goals

Setting goals is a very important aspect of making any modifications in your life. Setting goals is similar to having an action plan that you will follow to make changes. An action play can be a verbal or written agreement (with yourself) that you want to follow. If you develop an action plan, you will be more likely to be successful in making your change. Both your action plan and your goal should be as detailed and specific as possible. Though there are many ways to set goals, this chapter will review the SMART method (Table 1).

Table 1: The SMART method to setting and achieving goals

S	SPECIFIC	Set a *specific* simple behavior to change
M	MEASURABLE	Set up ways to *measure* your progress toward meeting your goal
A	ATTAINABLE	Make sure that your goal is *attainable*, and find ways to *achieve* your goal
R	REALISTIC	Make sure that your goal is *realistic*
T	TIMELY	Set up a *timeframe* for your goal so that you have a clear target

You have to be confident that you can achieve your goal; otherwise, you are setting yourself up for setbacks or even failure. If your goal is realistic and attainable, you should feel confident that you can achieve it in the time you allotted for yourself. Once you have set a goal, ask yourself "How confident am I that I will achieve this goal?" If the answer is lower then 85%, then you should consider resetting your goal so that it falls into at least a 90% confidence level. (See Charts 3 and 4 for examples of a completed SMART plan and a blank chart for you to use in setting your goals.

Once you have a specific goal that is realistic for you and that you are confident you can achieve, it may help to

Chart 3

Chart using the SMART method to set goals, including concerns and supports related to achieving those goals

General goal	Specific goal	Measurable	Attainable/confidence	Timely	My Concerns	My supports
To eat less junk food	I will eat healthy snacks (fruit, vegetables, low-fat foods)	3 times a day	90% confident	I will complete this in 3 weeks	I love cookies and brownies, and fruits and veggies are expensive.	My husband and coworker, Margie

Chart 4
Blank chart to use in setting goals with the SMART method

General goal	Specific goal	Measurable	Attainable/confidence	Timely	My Concerns	My supports

track your progress. Keeping a diary to measure your successes (or even failures) can be beneficial because you will be able to visualize what worked and what didn't. Also, sharing your goal or goals with someone else is a good way of ensuring that you will work on the goals.

Once we say our goal out loud, it becomes real. In sharing your goal, you can tell people specifically how they can support you. For example, if you want to go to the gym 3 times a week, but you know that you may need a ride sometimes or specific encouragement or incentives, ask someone to help you in these ways.

Your turn

Write down a goal that you want to accomplish

_____

Set Goals
- Setting goals gives you an action plan to follow
- Use SMART goals
    - Specific, measurable, attainable, realistic, timely
- Make goals as specific and detailed as possible
- Be confident that you will achieve your goal
- Track your progress

Action plan

Once you have a goal, you need to implement it. A good way to reach your goals and keep on track is to develop an action plan. An action plan includes the steps that will lead you to your goal. These will include a timeline, the supports you need, any environmental changes you need to implement, any new tools you need to acquire, etc. For example, if my goal is to eat healthy snacks in 3 weeks, my action plan may look like the one pictured in Chart 5. Try it yourself! Chart 6 is set up so that you can use it to identify the steps—your action plan—that you need to undertake to achieve your goals.

Don't give up

When you are trying to change, it is not uncommon to reach a point at which you want to give up. When you don't see progress right away, or when progress slows—as it inevitably will—frustration can set in. However, long-lasting changes are made gradually and take time and effort (up to 6 months to become a new habit). Changing your lifestyle starts by changing the way you think. But, the way you think is as ingrained and habitual (and as resistant to change) as your habit of biting your nails or cracking your fingers. Because of this, learning something new—such as a new behavior—requires much repetition. Do not give up after a short time; it is possible that your change hasn't become ingrained in your brain yet. Keep repeating your new behavior or behaviors, and they will become more automatic for both your body and your mind. Don't be too hard on yourself, and definitely don't give up! This is when your support system (family, friends, therapists, or even doctors) will come in handy. They can be crucial in helping you to stay on track, keep up your confidence, and accomplish your goals. It is also a good technique to identify the "red flags" that may indicate that you are slipping into old habits again. For instance, in trying to eat healthier, you may identify as red flags that, when you have are stressed, you want to grab the candy bar or, when you slip once, you tell yourself you've blown

Chart 5
Example of a completed chart to lay out the steps, supports, barriers, and solutions to reaching goals

Step	Supports	Barriers	Solutions
By (date), I will have identified 3 healthy snacks	I will buy the snacks and have them in my house in 4 days	I don't know what is healthy I can't get to the grocery store	I will do research online or ask to see a nutritionist I will ask someone to buy the snacks for me
By (date), I will have replaced 2 of my usual snacks with healthy snacks	I will do this on Tuesday and Thursday	I forget to bring them to work with me	I will find an alternative healthy snack in the vending machine, keep healthy snacks in my office, go out and get a healthy snack
By (date), I will have identified healthy drinks	I will buy the healthy drinks and have them in my house	I don't know what is healthy I need my coffee to keep me going I can't get to the grocery store	I will do research or ask a nutritionist I will decrease my coffee by one cup a week I will ask someone to go to the store
By (date), I will drink a healthy drink in place of my usual drinks 50% of the time	I will do this on Tuesday and Thursday when I eat my healthy snacks	I crave sugar I won't like it	I will post a sign in my office to encourage me to stick to my goals I will tell one coworker for support

Chart 6

Blank chart to lay out the steps, supports, barriers, and solutions to reaching my goals

Step	Supports	Barriers	Solutions

it all and eat junk foods. Identifying these flags and then planning how to overcome them will help you to keep you on track.

Don't Give Up!
- The best changes are made gradually and take time and effort
- Changes require a lot of repetition
- Patience is important
- You may experience setbacks—but don't be hard on yourself if you do have a setback
- Get support from family and friends

You aren't alone

While you are making changes, it is important to keep in mind those individuals in your life who can provide you with support. Friends, family members, and medical professionals can help you to implement changes as well as keep you on track with your routine. You can rely on these support systems to ask for help with your daily responsi-

---

You Aren't Alone
- Find a supportive network of individuals such as family members, friends, and health-care professionals
- Explain changes to others; this will help further facilitate change and maintain changes that you are making and will make
- Find others to help with your responsibilities so that you do not fatigue easily

---

bilities when you are hoping to delegate tasks to others so that you are not overwhelmed with responsibilities in your daily routine. Also, make others aware of the changes you are trying to incorporate into your life. When others are aware of why and how you are making changes, they will support you, your hard work, and your accomplishments throughout the whole process.

Summary

Now you know what will make the changes in your behavior stick. Make sure to not try to change too much at once. If you start with small changes, you will be more likely to accomplish these changes, and your confidence will increase. After you incorporate a few smaller changes into your life, incorporating more changes will seem easier. If you have friends and family members who support you, not only your changes, but also your accomplishments, will be more successful.

If you have completed each chapter, you have learned a method for managing your fatigue that you can use for the rest of your life. You will find that your way of thinking changes so that, when a new symptom appears or you experience a change in your multiple sclerosis, you will feel more confident in being able to adapt. If you added only one thing to your routine, like regular exercise or restoration to your day, then you have taken an important step in fighting your fatigue and being in control of your life.

INDEX